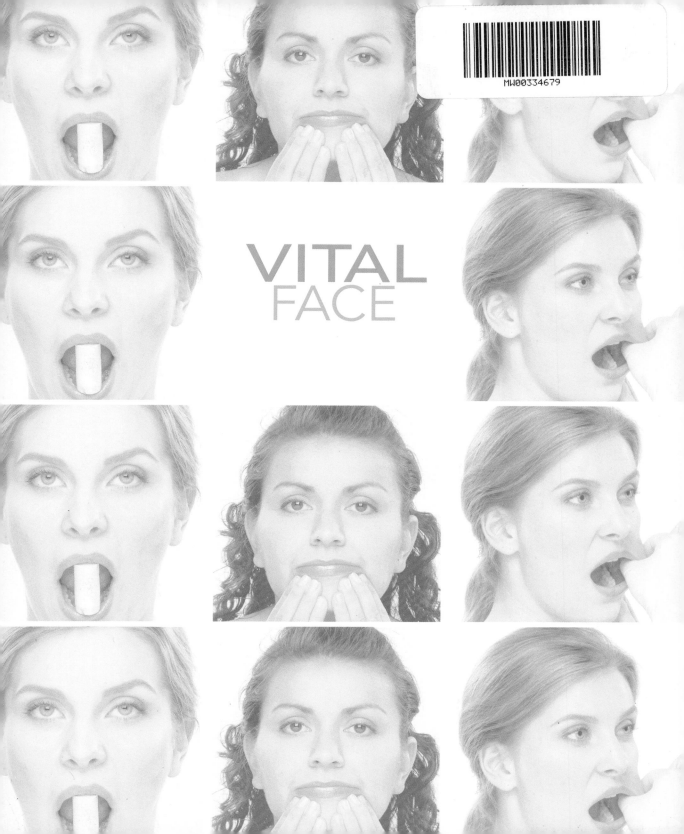

VITAL
FACE

This revised and enlarged English translation of Kasvot kuntoon. Kohenna kasvojesi terveyttä ja ulkonäköä was first published in Finland in 2009 by Otava Publishing Company Ltd

English language edition first published in 2013
by Singing Dragon
an imprint of Jessica Kingsley Publishers
73 Collier Street
London N1 9BE, UK
and
400 Market Street, Suite 400
Philadelphia, PA 19106, USA

www.singingdragon.com

Library of Congress Cataloging in Publication Data
A CIP catalog record for this book is available from the Library of Congress

British Library Cataloguing in Publication Data
A CIP catalogue record for this book is available from the British Library

ISBN 978 1 84819 166 2
eISBN 978 0 85701 130 5

Printed and bound in Canada

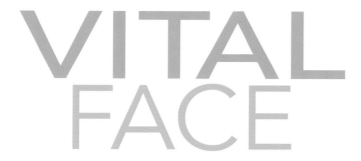

VITAL FACE

FACIAL EXERCISES AND MASSAGE FOR HEALTH AND BEAUTY

LEENA KIVILUOMA

PHOTOGRAPHS AND ILLUSTRATIONS BY RISTO KURKINEN

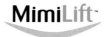

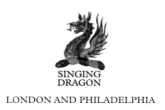

SINGING DRAGON

LONDON AND PHILADELPHIA

CONTENTS

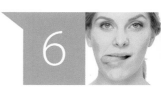

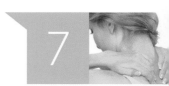

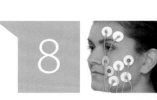

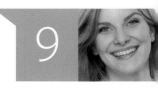

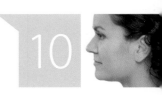

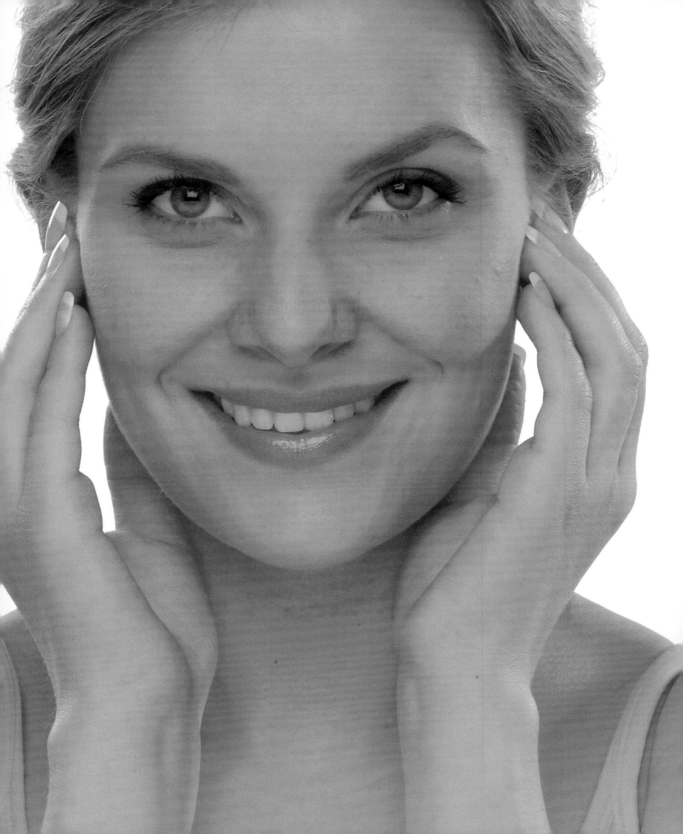

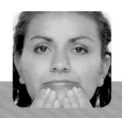

INTRODUCTION TO
MIMILIFT FACIAL
MUSCLECARE

1

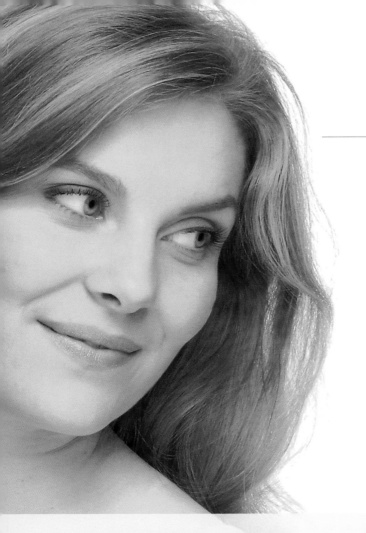

WHAT IS MIMILIFT FACIAL MUSCLECARE?

Muscles impact on both the health and appearance of the face as well as of the whole body. The facial muscles can be treated just like the other muscles of the body.

There are over 50 muscles in the facial area including both mimic muscles and chewing muscles on both halves of the face. These muscles get tense and tighten or weaken and get flabby like any other muscles in the body. The face feels tense and taut, the jaw becomes stiff and sore, and a headache is a common symptom. Lines and creases on the forehead and around the eyes and mouth get more visible and increase in number, facial volume decreases and facial features sag.

With the help of this book you will be able to treat these and many other muscle-based health problems and age-related changes in the facial region. This book presents an effective and safe programme for the muscles of the facial area, called **MimiLift Facial MuscleCare™**.

MimiLift Facial MuscleCare is a medical based system, developed by **Leena Kiviluoma**, a Finnish

WHO WILL BENEFIT FROM MIMILIFT?

1 **Anyone who has a stressed and tight feeling on her/his face**

Tensions of the facial region are reflected in the whole body. Relaxation of the face comprehensively relaxes the whole body, promotes wellbeing and helps falling asleep.

2 **Anyone interested in improving their appearance naturally**

The facial muscles have an important role in the appearance of the face. MimiLift Facial MuscleCare smooths out the facial lines and wrinkles and decreases their formation by relaxing the mimic muscles. The right training

techniques lift and fill the face by improving the condition, construction and elasticity of the facial muscles and ligaments. MimiLift Facial MuscleCare also improves the condition and appearance of the skin by stimulating the cells producing elastin and collagen and by stimulating blood circulation and lymphatic flow in the facial area.

3 **Those suffering from muscle-based headaches and facial pain**

Muscle-based headaches and facial pain are common problems. Headache is a symptom that almost everyone experiences every now and then, and muscle tension headache is the most common type of headache. Statistically about half of the population every once in a while

physiotherapist engaged in teaching and expert consultation in the fitness and rehabilitation industry. Recent research in many branches of medical science supports the theory and practical instructions of MimiLift Facial MuscleCare.

The programme consists of precise stretching and massage techniques and relaxing and strengthening exercises aimed at the mimic and chewing muscles. These procedures will improve both your health and the physical appearance of your face. Instructions for the maintenance of other muscles of the head and neck-shoulder region included in this book complement MimiLift Facial MuscleCare procedures and their effects are clearly explained.

You can easily choose just the right programme for your individual situation, needs and goals. MimiLift Facial MuscleCare gives you an opportunity to become actively involved in your own health and beauty care, giving you control over your own body.

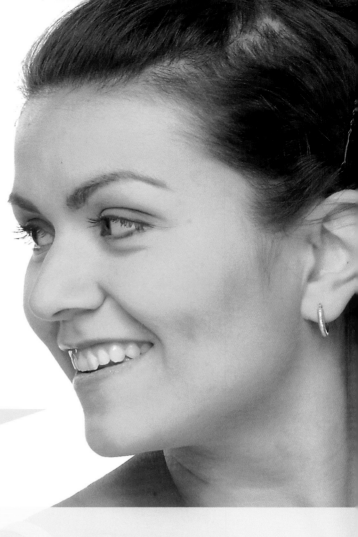

> This book presents a comprehensive and medical-based programme called **MimiLift Facial MuscleCare.**
>
> Every procedure of MimiLift Facial MuscleCare improves both health and facial appearance.

suffers from tension headache or facial pain. Often these problems can be eased, or even avoided, by relaxation of the mimic and chewing muscles.

4 Those who grind and clench their teeth

It is a common habit to grind, gnash or clench one's teeth unnecessarily and often unconsciously. People can clench their teeth while awake or during sleep. The chewing muscles will overload and get sore. The lower jaw feels stiff and the head is aching.

Teeth grinding, medically called bruxism, is a part of a larger group of symptoms and problems called temporomandibular disorders. Therefore, care of the chewing muscles is very important, both in preventive and therapeutic situations.

5 Those with pain in the neck-shoulder region

Soreness and tension in the chewing muscles spread easily into the neck-shoulder region and vice versa. Collapsed upper body posture is a common postural problem which in the long term can easily result in pain in the neck-shoulder and facial regions. Posture correction prevents muscle tightness and nerve entrapment syndromes, thus contributing to the welfare of the face, neck and shoulders.

6 Speakers, lecturers, teachers, actors and singers

Teachers, actors, singers, speakers, sales people and other people in customer service use their voice a lot in their work. For them, their voice is often their most

WHAT IS MIMILIFT USED FOR?

HEALTH · WELLBEING · INTERACTION · VOICE PRODUCTION

- relaxes the face
- relaxes the whole body
- reduces and prevents tension headache and facial pain
- reduces stiffness of the lower jaw
- relieves the voice muscles for better speaking and singing
- increases self-awareness of facial expressions and habits
- promotes positive interaction and communication
- improves posture and eases neck and shoulders
- helps in rehabilitation of bite disorders

APPEARANCE
Smooths out

- horizontal forehead creases
- furrows between the eyebrows
- lines around the eyes and mouth
- nose-to-mouth furrows
- horizontal chin creases

- makes cheeks and lips fuller
- lowers nose-to-mouth fold
- decreases folds and lines on the neck
- tones neck
- gives face a healthy glow
- reduces facial puffiness
- stimulates renewing of facial skin

valuable tool. Speaking and singing require the work of muscles. Chewing muscles move the lower jaw, and the mimic muscles and the muscles of the tongue are involved in voice production. Relaxed and stressless voice production needs to be supported by correctly working muscles.

MimiLift Facial MuscleCare decreases stress, stiffness and tightness of the voice-producing muscles. For example, the right kind of maintenance of facial and voice-producing muscles will enable actors to relax and prepare themselves for the spontaneous emotional expression of the character they are playing. With the help of the same technique, they are able to free their face and voice from the playing the role.

7 Professionals in sales and marketing

Facial expressions and tone of the voice play an important role in the interaction between human beings. A relaxed face and pleasant voice in business communication situations, as well as in private life, give a positive impression to the person you are communicating with.

8 Violinists and wind instrument players

Playing any wind instrument or playing violin or viola may cause unusually high stress in the facial area of the musician. Musicians who play wind instruments often have problems with the chewing muscles and mimic muscles around the mouth and cheeks. According to recent research, over 70% of violinists suffer from stress, tension and stiffness of the chewing muscles and have

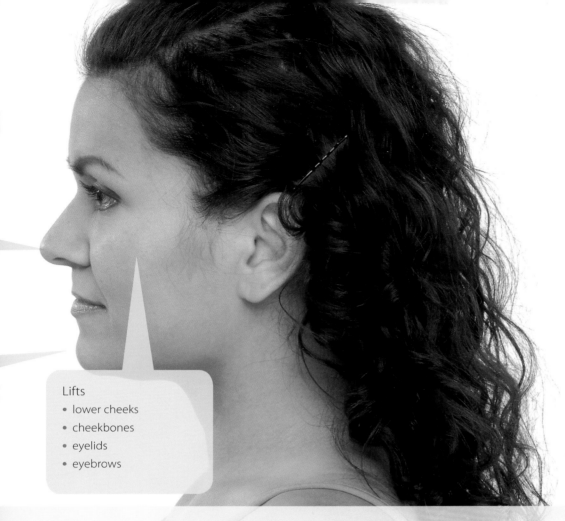

Lifts
- lower cheeks
- cheekbones
- eyelids
- eyebrows

problems with their jaw joints. The reason for this is the playing position where the instrument is supported asymmetrically under one half of the lower jaw. This puts the lower facial muscles and the jaw joints under a lot of stress. Massage and stretching techniques of the chewing and mimic muscles and neck and shoulders will help the body to recover from the stress caused by playing.

9 Dancers and athletes in aesthetic sports

Dance, figure skating and rhythmic gymnastics are aesthetic sports. Stiffness and tension in one part of the body will be reflected in other parts of the body. Stress and tension in the facial area will easily transfer to the upper body, harming the general impression and feeling of a relaxed and free presentation. A relaxed face with a free, natural expression will support the enjoyable artistic performance.

10 Bell's palsy patients and other patient groups

Dysfunction or trauma of the facial nerve results in lack of movement of the mimic muscles. The rehabilitation of Bell's palsy includes restoring normal nerve-muscle function of the mimic muscles by specific exercises and programmes planned specifically for the situation.

Many illnesses that impact muscles and nerves in any part of the body may have also an impact on the muscles and nerves of the face. Among these are stroke, Parkinson's disease and multiple sclerosis (MS). It is possible to use MimiLift Facial MuscleCare in the rehabilitation of those suffering from these illnesses. However, the most suitable individual procedures should be chosen with the health care professionals treating the patient.

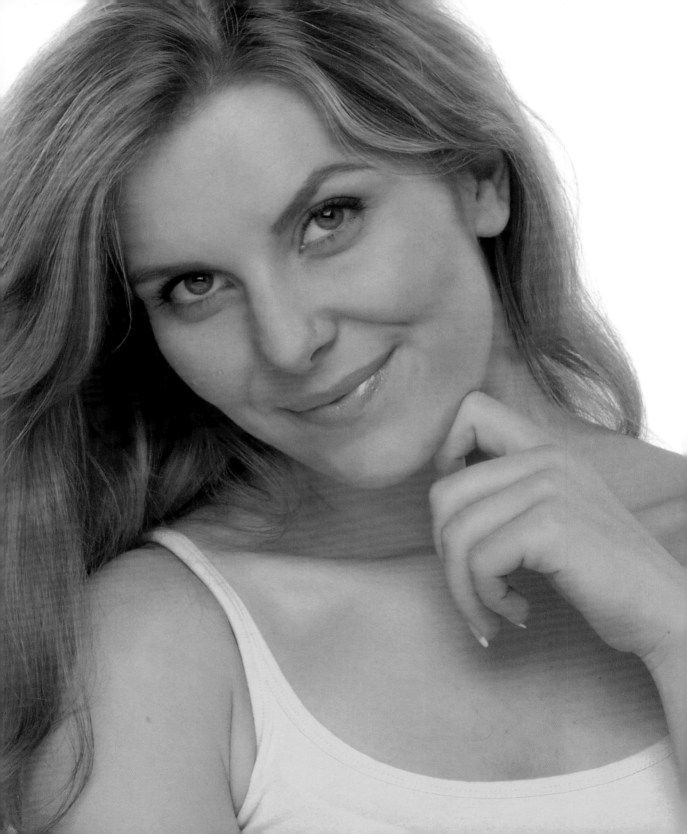

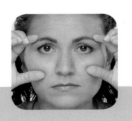

ANATOMY
AND PHYSIOLOGY
OF THE FACE

2

STRUCTURE AND FUNCTION
OF THE MIMIC AND CHEWING MUSCLES

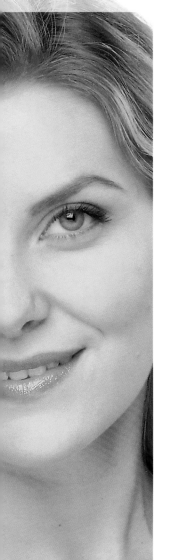

The muscular system does not end at the neck, but covers all of the head. The structure of the muscles in the facial area corresponds to that of other voluntary muscles in the body which are responsible for initiating motion. The chewing muscles and mimic muscles are part of the whole musculoskeletal system of the body.

Size, number and type of muscle cells

The mimic and chewing muscles are voluntary, striated, skeletal muscles of the body. Voluntary means that you are able to control what these muscles do – for example, your jaw does not open to bite an apple unless you want it to open. Skeletal muscles are also called striated muscles because under the microscope the light and dark parts of the muscle cells appear to look striated.

Similar to other skeletal muscles, mimic and chewing muscles are composed of thin, elongated cylindrical muscle cells also known as muscle fibres. One muscle is made up of many muscle cells running all the way from the origin to insertion. Thousands of muscle cells together make up the entire muscle.

The individual muscle cells in the mimic muscles are smaller than those in the chewing muscles or in the other larger skeletal muscles. The mimic muscles are small and weak compared to the chewing muscles and strong limb muscles, not only due to their smaller cell size, but also because the total number of muscle cells in mimic muscles is much smaller. For example, zygomaticus major, one of the mimic muscles, may contain about 6000 muscle cells, whereas biceps brachii, a muscle of the upper limb, may contain about 300,000 muscle cells.

Two types of muscle cells are found in skeletal muscles: slow-twitch cells and fast-twitch cells. All muscles contain a mixture of these cells. The higher the number of fast-twitch cells, the faster the muscle can contract. A calf muscle contains about 20% fast-twitch cells and the ring muscle of the eye about 85%, which shows that eye blinking requires a lot of speed.

Building materials of muscles

Each muscle cell is full of protein-rich filaments called actin and myosin filaments that are arranged length-wise in the muscle. The muscle contracts when actin and myosin filaments interact by sliding deeply between each other. Strength training increases the amount of these contractile proteins. This increases the size of muscle cells and adds volume to the muscle.

The soft muscle tissue is supported by connective tissue made of collagen and elastin. A connective tissue surrounds individual muscle cells. The muscle cells are

STRONG AND PLUMP FACIAL MUSCLES

The strengthening exercises of MimiLift Facial MuscleCare challenge the muscles of the facial area to perform the movements effectively in the widest possible range of motion available to them. This means that increasingly more motor units in the facial muscles are activated, which in turn builds the proportion of active muscle tissue. With the size of the individual muscle cells in the muscles increasing, facial muscularity becomes stronger and plumper.

The procedures of MimiLift Facial MuscleCare also strengthen and remould the facial fascias and ligaments. Strong yet elastic facial fascias and ligaments together with firm, well-conditioned facial musculature reduce facial sag and create a perfect natural facelift.

RELAXED FACIAL MUSCLES

Unpleasant and harmful muscle tightness and tension in the facial area can be relieved by the unique massage and stretching techniques of MimiLift Facial MuscleCare. These relaxing procedures penetrate the surface of the skin, thus remoulding the underlying muscles. They apply multidirectional stretching to the cells of taut muscles, relieving muscle stiffness.

MimiLift Facial MuscleCare releases tension in the whole facial myofascial system. Facial relaxation is vital for facial health by eliminating muscle-based facial pains and headaches.

Relaxed mimic and chewing muscles that retain their normal length and tone make facial features soft, giving the face a peaceful, pleasant look.

Relaxation of the mimic muscles smooths out lines and creases. MimiLift Facial MuscleCare is a totally non-invasive line-smoothing method.

arranged in bundles and these bundles are wrapped in a connective tissue covering called fascia. Besides having a supportive function, the connective tissue brings elasticity to the muscles.

Mimic muscles are not enveloped by such definite fascias as other skeletal muscles. In the facial area a fibrous sheet of varying degrees of thickness envelops the facial musculature and thus connects the mimic muscles for coordination of facial expressions.

Mimic muscles are connected partly to the facial bones and partly straight to the facial skin with a fibrous network and several retaining ligaments. Connective tissues also attach the chewing muscles to the bones of the head.

Motor unit of muscle cells

One motor nerve plus all the muscle cells it activates is called a motor unit. The fewer muscle cells there are per motor unit, the more accurate the control of the nerves over a muscle. In the facial muscles, a single motor nerve activates only a few muscle cells because facial muscle action requires fine-motor skills to produce high-precision movements that require little strength. In contrast, in muscles of the limbs that contribute to force production, a single motor nerve can send impulses to several hundreds or even thousands of muscle cells at a time.

The muscle cells of a single motor unit are not arranged side by side in a muscle but dispersed between the muscle cells of other motor units. When motor units are activated, muscle contraction is generated evenly in the muscle and the performance of movement becomes smooth. The contraction of single motor cells follows the principle of 'all or nothing'. In other words, muscle cells cannot choose to contract separately at half load or full load but always contract at full load. Regulation of muscle force is based on the number of motor units recruited. When more force or larger movements are needed, the impact of each motor unit becomes greater so more motor units are activated.

Muscle tonus

Even at rest, most of our skeletal muscles are not completely switched off. They are in a state of a partial contraction called tonus. A resting muscle is not totally flaccid because a small set of motor units is constantly active to maintain the tonus. When one set of motor units relaxes, another set continues. Tensed muscle is a muscle with increased tonus, meaning more motor units are switched on.

FACIAL **NERVOUS SYSTEM**

The head office of facial muscle work and facial sensations is the brain. The brain sends and receives messages, which are carried through the nerves. The facial nerve is the motor nerve of mimic muscles. The trigeminal nerve is both the motor nerve of chewing muscles and the sensory nerve of the face.

Cranial nerves

The brain is the control centre of the whole body. Messages from the brain to the body and from the body to the brain are sent through the nerves. There are two kind of nerve fibres: motor and sensory fibres. Motor nerve fibres send signals to the muscles to move. Sensory nerve fibres send information about touch, pain and other sensory information from the body to the brain.

The nerves emerging directly from the brain are called cranial nerves. The nerves branching out from the segments of spinal cord are spinal nerves. In total there are 12 pairs of cranial nerves, numbered according to their attachments to the brain. The nerves in the facial region are cranial nerves. The motor nerve of the mimic muscles is the seventh cranial nerve, the facial nerve. The sensory nerve of the face and the motor nerve of the chewing muscles is the fifth cranial nerve, the trigeminal nerve.

Five main branches of the facial nerve

1. Temporal branch
2. Zygomatic branch
3. Buccal branch
4. Mandibular branch
5. Cervical branch

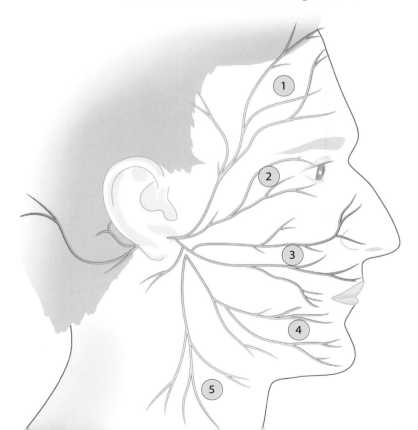

The facial nerve and the trigeminal nerve

The facial nerve originates in the bottom of the brain, separating into each side of the face and branching out to reach all the mimic muscles. The facial nerve has both motor and sensory fibres. The motor fibres of the facial nerve send signals to the mimic muscles to move. The sensory fibres of the facial nerve carry taste sensations from the front of the tongue.

The trigeminal nerve contains motor fibres which control the work of the chewing muscles, and sensory fibres which send information about touch, pain and temperature from the facial area to the brain. The trigeminal nerve has three major divisions emerging to the forehead and eye, cheek, and lower face and jaw. The motor fibres of the chewing muscles exist in the lowest nerve division, the mandibular division.

Voluntary and involuntary facial movements

The specific area of the brain responsible for controlling voluntary muscle movements is the motor cortex. Every part of the body occupies a particular region of the motor cortex which controls its movements. These delicate regions make up a kind of motor map of the body in the brain. On this map, the face occupies a notably large space, because the delicate, fine movements of mimic muscles demand much more control from the brain than, for example, flexing the knee. Furthermore, the lower part of the face takes up more space in this map than the upper part of the face, because the ability to use the region of the mouth for talking and eating is much more important than, for example, the ability to lift only one eyebrow.

We can usually control our facial movements at will, but not always. Strong emotions such as anger or fear cause involuntary facial expression in response. Involuntary facial movements appear because of the influence of the limbic system. The limbic system is an evolutionarily primitive brain structure which governs our emotions, particularly those that are related to survival.

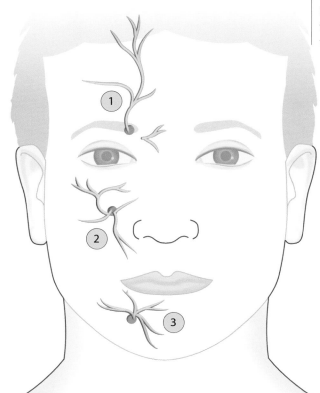

Three major divisions of the trigeminal nerve

1. Ophthalmic division
2. Maxillary division
3. Mandibular division

IMPACTS OF MIMILIFT FACIAL MUSCLECARE

MimiLift Facial MuscleCare improves your awareness of your facial muscles, which translates into an enhanced ability to control voluntary actions in your face.

You will be more aware of the tensions you hold in your face, which enables you to avoid unnecessary straining of your face and unflattering facial expression patterns.

BLOOD CIRCULATION IN THE FACE

Blood circulation is a transport system made up of vessels that carry the blood. The face is served by an abundant vascular system. Arteries carry oxygen-rich and nutrient-rich blood to the facial tissues. Veins carry oxygen-poor blood away from the face. The smallest blood vessels, called capillaries, reach all the facial tissues.

Facial arteries

The heart pumps the blood at a high pressure to the arteries to be distributed all over the body. The external carotid artery is the major distributing vessel responsible for bringing the blood to the facial region. It divides into four groups of branches of which the facial artery is the main artery of the facial skin and mimic muscles, while the maxillary artery supplies the chewing muscles and the deeper structures of the face. Main arteries subdivide into many smaller vessels, arterioles, and finally into the tiniest blood vessels, the capillaries, which form a dense network to serve all the cells in the facial area.

The walls of the blood capillaries are very thin, enabling all essential substances for the cells such as oxygen, nutrients and hormones to pass through these walls and enter the surrounding tissues.

Facial veins

The vessels that transport the waste products are the veins. In the capillaries the waste products, such as carbon dioxide, are transferred from the facial tissues into the vessels to be carried away. Venous capillaries gradually turn into larger and larger veins. Facial veins follow the course of arteries.

Just like the arteries, the veins are large blood vessels, but their muscular walls are thinner and they have lower blood pressure. Unlike arteries, and in order to prevent backflow, the veins have small valves permitting the blood flow in one direction only.

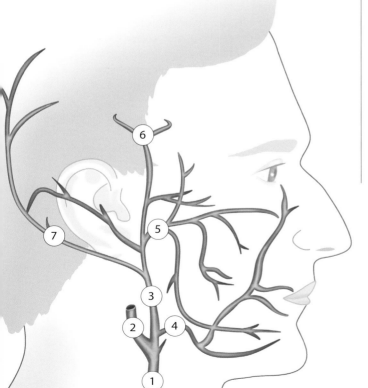

Facial arteries separating from the external carotid artery

1. Common carotid artery
2. Internal carotid artery
3. External carotid artery
4. Facial artery
5. Maxillary artery
6. Superficial temporal artery
7. Occipital artery

The blood returning from the head is assisted by gravity. The second aid is breathing which creates the changes in pressure within the thoracic cavity, thus propelling the venous blood back towards the heart. The third aid is muscle work. When we move and use our skeletal muscles, this creates a rhythmic pressure on the veins which helps the blood to flow.

Increased facial blood circulation

The capillaries can never all be open at the same time, because the total volume of blood in an adult human, about 5 litres, is not enough to fill all the vessels simultaneously. Blood is directed to the places where it is most needed. The capillaries open up and begin to conduct blood to the tissues and organs most in need of oxygen and nutrients. For example, when you begin to work your muscles, the capillaries in the muscles dilate and the blood flow to the muscles increases.

The increase of facial blood circulation means that resting capillaries in the facial region open up and the amount of blood flowing into the face increases. When the circulation increases in the numerous capillaries of the facial skin, the face turns red as the blood glows through the skin. The face reddens due to purely physiological reasons or due to emotional reasons. In the cheeks the capillaries are very near to the skin surface, and that is why the cheeks redden so easily.

Physiological flushing

The circulatory system helps the body to maintain its normal temperature by transporting heat. Your body and blood temperature rises during exercise. To help release this excess heat, more capillaries close to the skin will open. The blood transfers the heat to these capillaries, the heat of the blood warms your skin, and finally the excess heat is dissipated into the air. This is why your skin, especially your facial skin, turns a reddish colour when you are exercising.

The same thing happens because of outside factors. When the weather is hot, your blood vessels use the same method to keep the body's internal temperature at an even, normal level. The physiological function behind flushing is the enlargement of the capillaries in response to the nerves and various hormones activated by the autonomic nervous system.

Emotional blushing

Emotional blushing is an involuntary facial reddening due to emotional stimulation. It is visible in an area restricted to the face, ears, neck and upper chest.

You cannot decide whether to blush or not – it just happens. The walls of the blood vessels are smooth, involuntary muscles and you cannot control this type of muscle. It is the function of the motor neurons of the autonomic nervous system which can contract and relax capillaries. Nerve fibres involved in dilating the vessels of the face for blushing come from the nodules of the sympathetic nervous system, located in the thoracic spine.

IMPACTS OF MIMILIFT FACIAL MUSCLECARE

Facial massage, effective facial exercises and facial heat treatments increase the circulation locally in the facial area. Locally increased circulation from a massage helps to reduce facial muscle pains and headaches.

All the procedures of MimiLift Facial Muscle-Care boost circulation to the face. The delivery of essential nutrients and oxygen to the muscles and skin and all the other tissues of your face will improve.

The increased facial blood flow also carries more waste products away from the facial area. Increased facial blood circulation promotes cell renewal and a firmer skin with a healthy colour and glowing complexion.

LYMPHATIC DRAINAGE OF THE FACE

Lymphatic drainage is a network responsible for removing excess fluid and macromolecular waste products away from the tissues. The head and the neck contain many lymphatic vessels and nodes. A slowdown in the facial lymph flow may manifest as puffiness of the face.

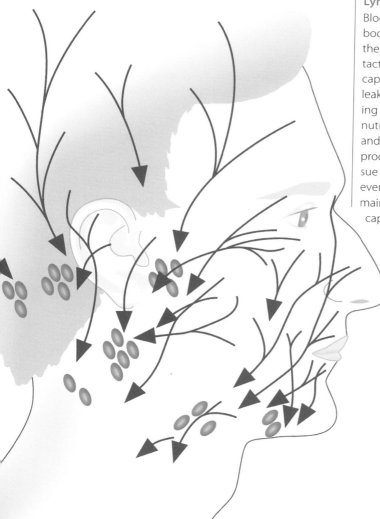

Lymphatic system

Blood transports essential materials around the body, but the blood itself does not come out from the blood vessels and does not come in direct contact with the body cells. When blood flows in the capillaries, it is a fluid similar to blood plasma that leaks through the capillary walls into the surrounding tissue. The fluid is called tissue fluid. It carries nutrients, oxygen, hormones and water to the cells and carries away carbon dioxide, nitrogenous waste products and water from the tissues. Most of the tissue fluid soon returns to the blood capillaries. However, a small amount remains outside, and this remaining fluid is sucked into a tiny tubes, lymphatic capillaries.

The tissue fluid that enters lymph capillaries is called lymph. Lymph fluid is transported back into blood circulation by a transporting system called lymphatic drainage. It is a drainage network made of lymph fluid, lymph vessels with one-way valves and lymph nodes.

Direction of the lymphatic drainage of the face and the scalp and some lymph nodes of the head

Facial lymphatic drainage

The facial area, as well as the whole head and neck, contains a lot of lymphatic vessels. The system of lymph vessels begins as close-ended lymph capillaries found in almost every tissue. The microscopic lymphatic capillaries unite to form larger lymph vessels. Eventually the lymphatic vessels converge into two ducts that empty the lymph fluid into the subclavian veins, which run beneath the collar bones. The lymph fluid goes back to the blood circulation and becomes blood plasma again.

Facial lymph flows only in one direction, from the facial tissues to the heart. Lymphatic drainage in the face generally follows the venous drainage.

Lymph nodes

Lymph nodes appear along the course of lymph vessels, and lymph flows through these nodes on its way back to the blood. Lymph nodes are small bean-shaped nodules made of small masses of lymphatic tissue. Lymph nodes are full of special cells called lymphosytes and macrophages, which filter and clean the lymph fluid before it enters the blood circulation.

Cleansing of the lymph is necessary for preventing the introduction of any harmful substances to the blood circulation. Since the walls of the lymph capillaries are flimsy, more thinner and more permeable than the walls of blood capillaries, bigger molecules which can not go into blood capillaries can enter lymph capillaries. That is why lymph fluid contains large protein molecules, fragments of dead cells as well as bacteria, viruses and other foreign materials which need to be destroyed.

Whenever bacteria and viruses try to attack the body, lymphosytes will rapidly multiply and the lymph nodes may become swollen, even painful. Sometimes in a medical examination a physician palpates the superficial lymph nodes found, for example, below your chin and running along the bottom of your jaw on both sides. Enlarged lymph nodes can reveal if there is an infection in your body. If the infection is mild, the node swelling will reduce as soon as the lymphatic system has destroyed the pathogens.

Improve your lymphatic flow

In the vascular system the heart functions as a pump, whereas lymph fluid is propelled by muscular action. Intrinsic muscle activity involves involuntary, intermittent contractions of the thin smooth muscle layer in the walls of lymphatic vessels. Extrinsic mechanisms include active use of the skeletal muscles, pressure changes in lungs associated with breathing and the help of gravity.

Lack of physical activity can lead to tissue swelling. Consequently, as waste products accumulate in the tissues, cells are less able to function properly, resulting in various metabolic and infectious problems. Chronic dehydration can also slow the flow of the lymph. The most important methods of promoting overall lymphatic circulation are exercise such as brisk walking and adequate hydration. In addition, facial lymphatic drainage is increased by proper face, head and neck massage and facial exercises.

IMPACTS OF MIMILIFT FACIAL MUSCLECARE

The procedures of MimiLift Facial MuscleCare stimulate lymph and blood circulation in the facial area, which reduces facial puffiness and is positively reflected in the condition of the facial skin.

BONES AND JOINTS OF THE FACE

The contour of the face primarily depends on the shape and dimensions of the underlying facial bone structure. The bones of the face provide attachment sites for the muscles and ligaments in the facial area. The only freely movable bone of the face is the lower jawbone, which articulates with the skull at the jaw joints.

Basis for the facial features

Bones contain both living cells and non-living minerals such as calcium. Bones are active tissue where osteoblast cells build new bone and osteoclast cells destroy old bone. The bones of the head are facial and cranial bones. They cushion and protect the brain and lay the basis for the facial soft tissues. In total, there are 22 facial and cranial bones joined together by immovable interlocking joints known as sutures.

The shape and dimensions of the facial bones largerly determine the features of the face. The zygomatic bone determines the height of the cheekbones, the shape of the lower jawbone is clearly reflected in the jaw angle and the chin, while the curvature of the forehead is shaped by the frontal bone.

Facial bone structure reveals sex and age

Differences in the facial bone structure are the main reason why the average female face differs from the average male face. Females seem to have slightly higher and more prominent cheekbones. Female chins are generally small and rounded with the jawline running in a graceful curve from the chin to the ear. Male jaws are more robust with more height, weight and prominence. Female noses are generally smaller, with a narrower and shorter nose bridge and a more refined nose tip. Male foreheads tend to be more sloping, with a prominent ridge on the frontal bone above the eye socket (brow ridge) whereas female foreheads are rounder with no brow ridge. However, it is the number of feminine or masculine features that makes a face look more female or male, not one particular feature.

Before puberty the facial features of boys and girls have no great differences, but they differ remarkably from the adult face. The face of a child is relatively flat, wide and vertically short. A child's forehead is large and slightly curved. The nose is small and short with a low nasal bridge. The lower jawbone is small and underdeveloped relative to the rest of the face.

Facial bones grow and develop gradually as a person matures. Facial bones keep changing throughout our lives, from infancy to old age, which is why adults never look quite the same as they looked in their early childhood.

Jaw joint (temporomandibular joint)

A joint is a place where two bones meet to allow a bone to move. The term temporomandibular refers to the connection between the temporal and mandibular bone. The jaw joints connect the jaw to the skull and let the lower jaw move up and down, sideways, forwards, backwards and in a circular motion. The jaw joint is formed by an outwards curving process of the lower jaw fitting into the inwards curving small cavity of the temporal bone.

Inside the jaw joint is an articular disc composed of dense fibrous connective tissue separating these two bones. As with any other joints, the jaw joints are supported by ligaments.

You can find the place of your jaw joint by placing your fingers gently just in front of your ears and moving your jaw up and down. What you are feeling under your fingers is the head of your lower jawbone moving.

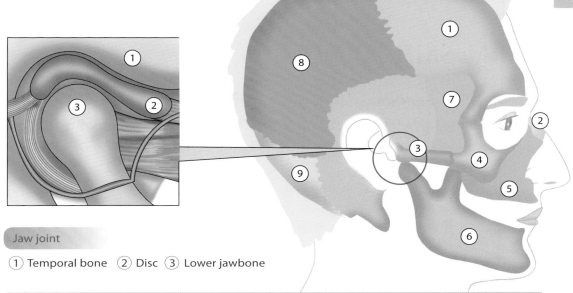

Jaw joint

(1) Temporal bone   (2) Disc   (3) Lower jawbone

BONES IN THE FACIAL REGION

(1) FRONTAL BONE

The frontal bone creates the region of forehead and provides the shape of the forehead. The portion in the centre of the frontal bone, between the eyebrows, is called the glabella.

(2) NASAL BONE

The nasal bone forms the root of the nose and the bridge of the nose. The tip of the nose is supported by tough, flexible connective tissue, nose cartilage.

(3) TEMPORAL BONE AND ZYGOMATIC ARCH

The temporal bone is located on the side of the head, above and behind the ear. The process of temporal bone projects to the facial area. It unites with the process of zygomatic bone. These two processes joined together form the whole zygomatic arch.

(4) ZYGOMATIC BONE

The zygomatic bone is a small bone below and lateral to the eye socket. It forms the prominence of the cheeks.

(5) MAXILLA (upper jawbone)

The maxilla is the bone of the mid-face. Maxilla holds the upper teeth. There are altogether 32 permanent teeth, 16 teeth in the upper jaw and another 16 in the lower jawbone.

(6) MANDIBLE (lower jawbone)

The mandible is the only freely movable bone of the head. It articulates with the skull at the temporomandibular joints (jaw joints). The shape of the mandible determines the jawline and the shape of mandible is clearly reflected in the jaw angle and chin.

OTHER BONES IN THE HEAD

(7) Sphenoid bone

(8) Parietal bone

(9) Occipital bone

IMPACTS OF MIMILIFT FACIAL MUSCLECARE

Bones need physical stress to remain strong. MimiLift Facial MuscleCare puts physical stress on facial bones through strengthening exercises and precise facial soft tissue manipulation techniques. These procedures stimulate the bone-building cells (osteoblasts) to grow new bone. Good facial bone density slows down age-related general facial bone shrinkage as well as changes of the bone shape, which prevents soft tissue sagging due to better bone support.

The procedures of MimiLift Facial MuscleCare reduce and prevent harmful pressure and faulty movements of the jaw joints and help them function in precise synchronized harmony.

FACIAL **SKIN**

Facial skin is composed of two layers, the epidermis and the dermis, which differ from each other in terms of structure and function. The thickness of the skin varies in different facial regions. The firmness and elasticity of the skin are largely dependent on the collagen and elastic fibres of the dermis.

Epidermis, the outer skin layer

The epidermis is a thin, tough outer layer of facial skin where there are no blood vessels. It is composed of several layers of epithelial cells, which serve to protect the underlying tissue like a coating.

The epidermis undergoes constant regeneration. The skin stem cells produce new daughter skin cells in the deep layers of the epidermis. As the stem cells keep reproducing new skin cells, the earlier produced daughter cells get pushed up toward the surface of the skin. During their journey they become flat and keratinized to form a protective barrier of layers of cells at the outermost surface of the epidermis (stratum corneum). The epithelial cells in the corneum

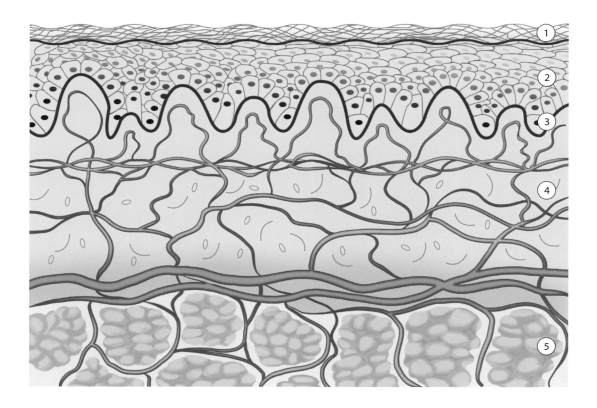

flake off about one month after creation and are continually replaced by inner cells moving outward.

The skin cells on the outermost surface are embedded in a matrix of lipids. Some of these lipids are synthesized in the epidermis whereas others are secreted on to the surface from the sebaceous glands. A well-functioning and well-lubricated epidermis protects the body from dehydration and external dangers. The acid mantle on the skin's surface is a combination of sebum and perspiration. The acid mantle with a normal, somewhat acidic skin pH inhibits the growth of foreign microorganisms.

When extra protection from ultraviolet rays is needed, specialized cells in the bottom of the epidermis begin to make a pigment called melanin. Melanin darkens the skin and filters out potentially harmful UV radiation from the sun.

The epidermis is tightly connected to the dermis by an elaborate connective structure, called the basement membrane. It differentiates the epidermal cells from the underlying dermis. The epidermis forms an undulating appearance, with intermittent regular protusions of the epidermis into the upper layers of dermis.

Dermis, the inner skin layer

Directly below the epidermis lies the dermis. The basic structure of the dermis is composed of collagen and elastic fibres and a gel-like ground substance. Collagen is a fibrous protein that gives the skin its form and strength, while elastic fibres give the skin its elasticity or spring. These fibres are bound together by ground substance. The water-binding ground substance made of amino sugar molecules (glycosaminoglycans) – for example, hyaluronic acid – gives skin its plumpness.

The dermis contains a dense network of blood vessels. The cells at the bottom of the epidermis receive the nutrients and oxygen needed for cell renewal by diffusing from the blood capillaries extending to the upper dermis. Because the junction between epidermis and dermis, known as the dermal-epidermal junction, is undulating, the surface area of the epidermis that is exposed to the capillaries is increased.

The dermis also contains hair follicles, oil and sweat glands and sense organs that detect touch, temperature and pain. The fibroblast are the stem cells of the dermis which produce new collagen, elastin and ground substance.

The dermis blends into the underlying hypodermis (subcutaneous tissue, or subcutis) without a distinct border.

FACIAL SKIN ANATOMY

(1) **STRATUM CORNEUM** is the outermost layer of epidermis – the skin layer you can see and touch.

(2) **EPIDERMIS** is composed of several layers of epithelial cells, which serve the underlying tissues like a coating.

(3) **DERMAL-EPIDERMAL JUNCTION** is a semipermeable barrier between the epidermis and dermis.

(4) **DERMIS** consists mainly of collagen and elastic fibres floating in a glycoprotein gel. Collagen provides skin with its strength and elastin provides it with flexibility. The dermis contains blood vessels, glands and nerve endings.

(5) **HYPODERMIS** is made of fat cells, which provide a layer of cushioning and insulation.

Superficial facial muscles are situated just under the skin. Usually muscles travel over joints, are connected to bones and put different parts of the the body in motion when contracting. The face is the only part of the body where one end of a muscle is not attached to a bone but straight to the skin. When the mimic muscles contract, they cause the overlying skin to move and the face to make expressions.

Hypodermis, the underskin

The hypodermis lies under the dermis, but it is not considered as a skin layer. The hypodermis is composed of fat cells and loose connective tissue. Fat cells have thin membranes enmeshed in a fibrous network. Without the supporting fibres, the fat cells would break down. The supporting network of connective tissue divides fat cells into a lobules. Besides supporting action for the fat cells, the connective tissue contains blood and lymph vessels and nerves.

Subcutaneous fat varies greatly in thickness among individuals and in different regions of the face. It is

SURFACE ANATOMY OF THE FACE

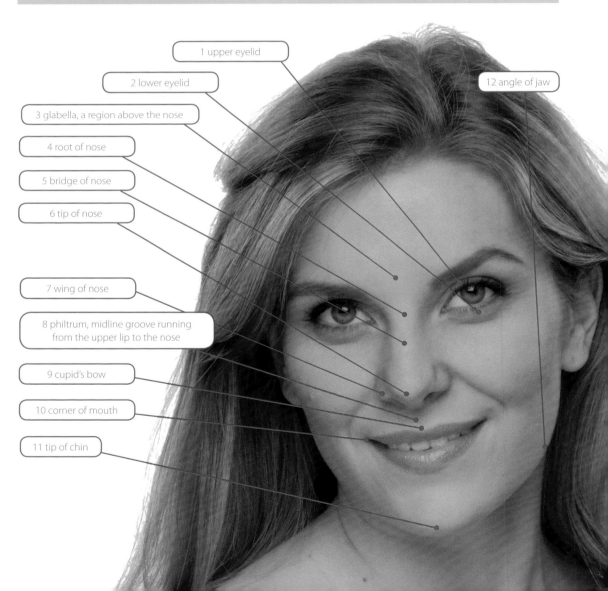

1 upper eyelid

2 lower eyelid

12 angle of jaw

3 glabella, a region above the nose

4 root of nose

5 bridge of nose

6 tip of nose

7 wing of nose

8 philtrum, midline groove running from the upper lip to the nose

9 cupid's bow

10 corner of mouth

11 tip of chin

the thickest in the cheeks. Fat cells are found abundantly in the fat pads of the cheeks, which are responsible for giving roundness especially to children's cheeks. Facial fat provides insulation and padding.

Under the hypodermis lie the muscles. A fibrous network with several retaining ligaments which emanate from the dermis connect the facial skin straight to the underlying mimic muscles. That is why a contraction of mimic muscles can move the facial skin and create expressions.

Chewing muscles, like all the other skeletal muscles of the body, have no straight connections to the skin. Skeletal muscles are connected to the bones and put the body in motion. That is why chewing muscles move the lower jawbone, not the facial skin.

Facial skin thickness

The thickness of the facial skin – epidermis and dermis together – is about 2.5 mm, from which the dermis makes up about 90%. Facial skin thickness varies considerably depending on sex and age but also between different regions of the face. Skin thickness is significantly greater on the tip of the nose and chin than on the forehead and cheeks. The upper eyelid has the thinnest skin.

There are no obvious differences in thickness of the skin in the same region between young boys and girls. In adolescents, due to hormonal influences, the male skin is characteristically thicker than female skin in all anatomic regions. Male hormones yield a denser network of collagen and elastic fibres than found in the female skin. In addition, the presence of terminal hair follicles results in thicker facial skin in men.

Thinning of the facial skin is a characteristic aspect of age-related changes, known as chronological ageing. As we grow old, the stem cells in the bottom of epidermis produce fewer and smaller new skin cells than before. The outer skin layer becomes thinner, even though the number of cell layers remains unchanged. The dermis, the inner skin layer, becomes thinner because aged fibroblast produce less collagen, elastin and ground substance. Changes in the dermis play a big role in the chronological ageing of the skin.

IMPACTS OF MIMILIFT FACIAL MUSCLECARE

The manual soft tissue techniques of MimiLift Facial MuscleCare stimulate fibroblast activity in the skin, boosting the skin's natural collagen and elastin production.

MimiLift Facial MuscleCare stimulates blood circulation in the facial capillaries. Improved circulation enhances the supply of oxygen and nutrients to the renewing skin cells. The result is youthful, glowing skin.

FACIAL **MUSCLES** AND **EMOTIONS**

E motions are connected to the face. Emotions are conveyed from one person to another through facial expressions. Different emotions activate different facial muscles, producing different facial expressions.

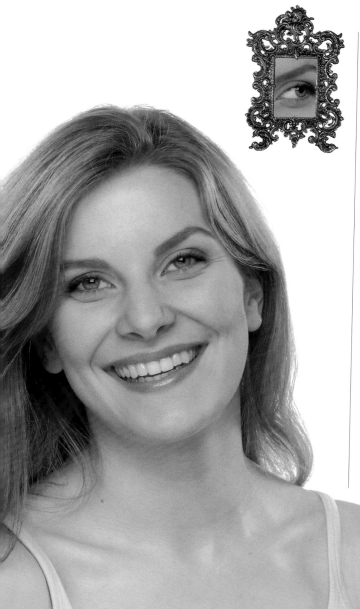

Genuine, involuntary facial expressions

Basic emotions help both human beings and other mammals to survive, adapt in the environment and reproduce. Their main role is to prepare the body to act quickly without conscious thought, to 'fight or flee'.

Basic emotions such as fear, anger, disgust, sadness, desire and joy produce differentiated facial muscle movements and facial expressions. For example, genuine, truly felt enjoyment automatically activates facial muscles expressing the signs of real joy.

Facial expressions of spontaneous, genuine emotions are governed by the limbic system. The limbic system is the evolutionarily primitive brain structure causing involuntary facial expressions in response to genuine, real emotions.

Because of their evolutionary survival function, genuine emotional reactions are elicited fast and last from a few seconds to a few minutes.

Spontaneous, genuine facial expressions are not learned, but are genetically coded in the brain of all human beings. Recent studies show that even congenitally blind individuals from different countries and cultures produce the same spontaneous, discrete facial expressions of emotion (Matsumoto, Willingham 2009).

Acted, voluntary facial expressions

In social interactions people often control their facial expressions. People who experience negative emotions may decide to smile to conceal their true feelings. False smiles and other acted, unfelt facial expressions are not produced by the limbic system. This kind of voluntary facial movement is produced by another pathway, by the specific area of the brain responsible for controlling all voluntary muscle movements, the area called the motor cortex.

A real smile automatically activates two facial muscles; in the cheek area the zygomatic major, which raises the corner of the mouth, and in the eye area, the orbicularis oculi, which forms the wrinkles to the corners of the eye. The unfelt, false smiles do not include activation of the orbicularis oculi muscles. In fact, it is difficult to create real-looking facial expressions voluntarily.

Even though people could mask their negative emotions behind voluntarily controlled facial expressions, a tiny involuntary microexpression can appear in their face for a very brief moment. Because this microexpression, lasting under a second, is produced by the limbic system, it can reveal the true emotions.

Facial expressions are contagious

Nonverbal expressions are the basis of interaction. Facial expressions of another person's genuine emotions are processed fast and automatically. When viewing a person with a genuine smile, the observation of a real, felt enjoyment evokes compatible facial muscle activity and compatible emotional experience in the observer. This is called emotional contagion. Observation of other people's emotions automatically evokes parallel expressions and experiences in the observers (Dimberg 1982, Surakka 1998, Surakka, Hietanen 1998). Real emotional facial expressions activate similar facial muscles and similar emotions much stronger than acted facial expressions.

Facial expressions of unpleasant emotions lead to greater emotional contagion than pleasant emotions. Hostility is transmitted from one person to another more easily than positive emotions. The stronger the emotional expression, the more susceptible the emotional contagion (Barsade, Sigal 2002). However, there are individual differences in

IMPACTS OF MIMILIFT FACIAL MUSCLECARE

With the help of MimiLift Facial MuscleCare you will develop an improved awareness of your facial muscles, which enables you to avoid unfavourable facial expression patterns.
MimiLift techiques release facial tensions and cause great overall relaxation.
A relaxed face with an enhanced awareness of the facial expressions improves nonverbal communication.

susceptibilty to emotional contagion.

In addition to facial expressions, in interaction people unconsciously mimic other kind of nonverbal expressions too, such as body postures and vocal utterances. Hearing vocal emotional expressions is contagious and activates facial muscles. For example, the muscles between the eyebrows, the frowning muscles, are activated more while hearing angry vocal sounds than content sounds.

Facial expressions and biochemical changes

Facial muscles are closely connected to emotions. Genuine emotions activate facial muscles and emotions transmit through facial expressions.

Research has also found that voluntary facial movements can turn on emotions. When people voluntarily activated the facial muscles used in smiling, it evoked positive emotions.

Basic emotional reactions cause chemical changes in the body in response. Positive emotions release 'feel-good' hormones giving a sense of well-being. Negative emotions release stress hormones, tense the muscles, raise the heart rate and blood pressure. Facial expressions have a great impact both on our mind and body, and our overall well-being and health.

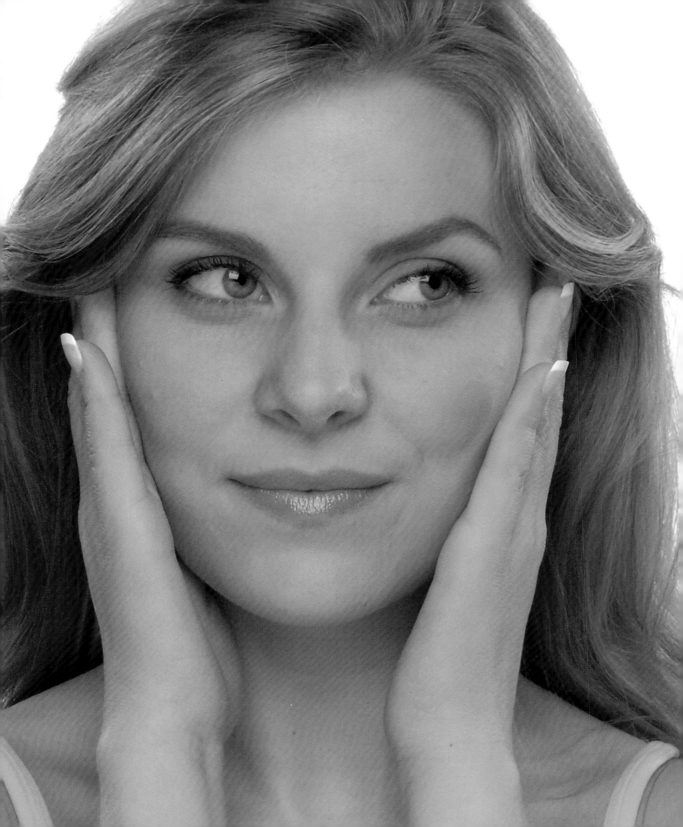

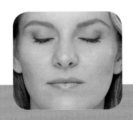

AGEING
FACE 3

THEORIES ON AGEING

Your calendar age does not tell your real age. Your real age is your biological age, the condition of your body's various tissues. Biological ageing is extremely individual due to genetic, environmental and lifestyle factors. There is no exact timetable to determine the rate and amount of changes that will result from ageing.

Distinguish chronological age from biological age

Ed Whitlock ran a marathon in less than three hours over the age of 70. Abdeslam Chellaf performed as an acrobat in a circus at the age of 65. In muscle strength measurements of large muscle groups, some 70-year-olds achieve the results that are typical at the age of 30.

Biological and chronological age are not the same. Chronological age is just a number and refers only to the numbers of years a person has lived. Our bodies are programmed to regenerate – repair, replace and protect our cells. Our body's ability to regenerate diminishes over time. Signs of biological ageing appear when the body regenerates more slowly than it degenerates. Biological age refers to the changes at the cellular and hormonal level. The rate of change varies individually due to genetic and lifestyle differences.

Your age should be judged based on biological factors rather than simply your year of birth. Your chronological age does not indicate the condition of the body's various tissues.

Your body is programmed to regenerate

Cells are the basic units of our body. All our tissues and organs are made up of cells, and all the processes of our bodies occur at the cellular level. Most cells in the human body regenerate within a certain period of time. Cells wear out, die naturally and new cells are produced to replace the lost cells. The cell division process that produces new cells for growth, repair and general replacement of older cells is the most important characteristic of a cell.

The cells that ensure a continuous supply of new cells to replace old cells that wear out or are destroyed are called stem cells. Stem cells exist almost everywhere in the body. Stem cells have been found, for example, in tissues such as the skin, skeletal muscles, bone marrow, blood, blood vessels and liver. The rates at which cells are replaced vary and depend on the type of the tissue. Tissues that undergo continuous turnover, such as skin, hair, fingernails, the stomach's protective lining and red blood cells, are replaced constantly at a rapid rate. Bones and muscles are replaced too, but the turnover time is longer.

Adult stem cells are capable of regenerating the human body for an amazingly long time and keep the body functioning properly and healthily throughout our lives. Chronological age really does not correlate with the biological age of most of your tissues.

Theories on ageing

Scientists have developed many theories to answer the questions 'Why do we age?' and 'How do we age?' Theories that explain how we age tell us the results of the biological ageing process. Based on these theories most of the us have heard that skin begins to wrinkle and thin, muscle and bone mass decreases, vision deteriorates and hearing becomes impaired.

Asking why we age has led scientists to investigate the nature of biological ageing itself. A critical issue in ageing research is whether ageing is affected by one, several or even hundreds of biological pathways. Complementary hypotheses include theories of telomere shortening, DNA damages, oxygen free radicals and glycation of tissues.

Glycation

Glycation is a process where glucose (sugar) molecules develop inappropiate attachments or cross-links to proteins. Glucose and protein tangle together much more readily if the amount of glucose in the blood is persistently higher than the normal, healthy level. Glycation makes tissues and organs stiff and inflexible, resulting in ageing in tissues where flexibility is most important, such as in the skin.

Oxygen free radicals

Oxygen free radicals are toxic byproducts of cell metabolism. These dangerous free radicals are neutralized by natural substances within our cells called antioxidants. Some free radicals escape this clean-up process and they can damage cells, especially cellular DNA. This oxidative damage accumulates over time. Oxidative damage is suggested to be one of the direct causes of ageing.

DNA damage

DNA damage happens throughout our lives. Spiral-shaped DNA molecules contain all the information a cell needs to sustain itself. These instructions are found in genes, which are sections of DNA. Mutations or spontaneous changes in the structure of the genes are continuously corrected and eliminated by enzymes called sirtuins.

If there is too much oxidative damage and too many harmful environmental factors such as x-rays, ultraviolet radiation and numerous toxic chemicals, sirtuins do not have enough time time to correct all the DNA damage. Mutations will accumulate, causing the cells to malfunction. This process has been suggested to be a crucial component in the ageing process.

Telomere shortening

Telomere shortening can be described as a sort of cellular clock that contributes to human ageing. Telomeres are appended as caps on the ends of all chromosomes in all of our cells and protect a cell's chromosomes from fusing with each other or rearranging. Each time a cell divides and a chromosome reproduces itself, a small bit of telomere is lost. Once telomeres become critically short, cells can no longer multiply to replenish body tissues. The cellular clock runs at different rates for different people. According to recent studies, this cellular clock can also run backward with the aid of enzyme that lengthens telomeres, named telomerase.

PREMATURE AGEING

Premature ageing means that the process of growing old is occuring at an accelerated rate. The changes in the body associated with ageing occur faster than they should do for the present age.

The first signs of premature ageing tend to appear in the face. Some of the worst things that causes premature ageing are:

- a diet containing too much sugary food and refined carbohydrates
- a diet low in proteins, essential fatty acids, vitamins and minerals
- excessive exposure to the sun
- smoking
- drinking too much alcohol
- lack of exercise
- too much negative stress

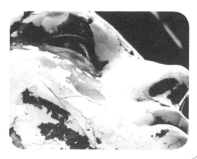

Bad lifestyle habits are an evident cause of premature ageing, which is good news, because you have the opportunity to influence the ageing process. We cannot stop ageing, but with many lifestyle choices we can slow down the biological ageing processes and experience as successful ageing as possible.

AGEING SKIN

Ageing changes in the skin including thinning, skin laxity, fragility and wrinkles are due to weakened cell function in the epidermis and dermis. Many of the changes are not natural ageing, but premature ageing caused by lifestyle choices. The most visible change is wrinkling of the skin which is caused by deterioration of structural components of the dermis.

Skin wrinkling

The structural framework of the skin is found in the dermis, where collagen and elastic fibres form a network to support the skin. Collagen gives skin its strength, and elastic fibres give the skin its elasticity. The effects of ageing are significant in this dermal layer of the skin. Collagen begins to deteriorate, less new collagen is produced and elastic fibres wear out. These changes cause the skin to wrinkle and become loose.

Skin thinning

With ageing, the stem cells in the bottom of epidermis produce fewer and smaller new skin cells. The outer skin layer becomes thinner, even though the number of cell layers remains unchanged.

In the dermis numerous fibroblast cells synthesize collagen, elastin and ground substance containing glycosaminoglycans such as hyaluronic acid. Ground substance has a gel-like consistency and it provides bulk, makes the skin plump, allowing the dermis to act as a shock absorber. Dermis thins because ageing fibroblast cells produce less collagen, elastin and ground substance.

Skin drying

Reproductive hormones stimulate oil-producing glands. As hormone levels fall, so does oil production, causing skin to become dry, itchy or flakey. Men experience a minimal decrease, but women's skin gradually produces less oil after the menopause.

The ground substance, especially hyaluronic acid, binds water and keeps the skin well hydrated. As the aged fibroblast cells produce less hyaluronic acid than younger fibroblast, there are fewer moisture-holding elements and the skin will dry.

Decrease of skin blood flow

A good blood flow is needed for proper cell function and regeneration. The epidermis contains no blood vessels, and the stem cells in bottom of the epidermis get their oxygen and nutrients by diffusion from the small blood vessels (capillaries) extending to the upper layers of the dermis. The junction between the dermis and epidermis interlocks, forming finger-like projections. These ridges increase the area of the blood capillaries.

As a person ages, the ridges of the dermal-epidermal junction flatten out. This process decreases the amount of nutrients available to the epidermis by decreasing the surface area in contact with the capillaries of the dermis. As the ageing skin receives less blood flow, the skin's normal regeneration and repair weakens.

Photoageing, smoking and alcohol

Everyone ages differently and the rate of changes in the skin varies markedly in individuals. Most of the 'ageing' of the skin is actually due to the effects of environment, not genetics. Lifestyle choices can speed up or slow down the process of skin ageing. The two worst environmental ageing factors are ultraviolet light and tobacco smoking.

Sun damage skin ageing, called photoageing, is a ultraviolet radiation injury to the layers of the skin. Repeated exposure to UV radiation breaks down dermal collagen, impairs new collagen synthesis and damages elastin fibres. Photoageing is characterized by wrinkles, dry and rough skin, mottled pigmentation and loss of skin tone. It is not only spending too much time in the sunlight that is harmful to the skin, but also UV tanning equipment which produce rays that cause premature wrinkling.

Ageing of the skin is accelerated by smoking. Long-term smokers have more facial wrinkles than non-smokers of the same age. Nicotine damages the collagen and elastin and weakens arteries. Smoking constricts blood vessels, reducing blood flow to the skin. Carbon monoxide takes the place of oxygen in the red blood cells. When skin cells are deprived of the nutrients and oxygen supplied by the blood, the skin wrinkles, thins out, loses its glow and becomes pale with an unhealthy grey tone.

Drinking too much alcohol also causes premature ageing. Alcohol contains ethanol, a toxin with many harmful effects on the body, including the skin. Excessive alcohol intake starves the body of the essential nutrients, including vitamins. For example, the depletion of the vitamins A and C supply decreases collagen production, reducing the thickness of the skin and causes wrinkles.

Poorly nourished skin

The third major factor is bad eating habits. Poor nutrition over a long period accelerates skin ageing. In particular, a low-protein and fat-free diet can have a devastating effect on the skin.

Protein is the basic building material of the collagen and elastic fibres in the dermis and the keratinocyte skin cells in the epidermis. The cells need protein to maintain their health, and protein is the main substance to replace the dead cells. With a lack of protein, the skin becomes thinner, loses elasticity and wrinkles.

Essential fatty acids are necessary to make skin cell membranes and to build epidermal lipids. A diet low in essential fatty acids makes the skin unable to retain its moisture. The skin becomes dry, characterized by a tight, rough feel and dull appearance.

Lifestyle affects more than genetics

Indentical twin studies have provided an excellent opportunity to compare genetics and environmental factors in the skin ageing process. Because the twins are identical genetically, any differences found were believed to result from external factors. Studies have shown that lifestyle choices have far more impact on skin ageing than the genetic inheritance.

Twins showing the greatest discrepancies in visible ageing signs also had the greatest differences between personal lifestyle choices and habits. Facial wrinkles were situated in the same area, but the number and depth of the wrinkles and the amount of skin laxity were significantly greater in siblings with a history of overexposure to sunlight and smoking. Other contributory lifestyle factors included excess alcohol consumption, poor diet and negative stress.

SAGGING FACIAL FEATURES

Facial ageing is not just the wrinkles seen in the skin's surface. Ageing affects all the tissues of the face. Age-related facial muscle, fat and bone atrophy (tissue wasting) leads to progressive facial volume loss. As volume decreases, the areas of the face deflate, soft tissues shift downwards and sagging and drooping increases.

Facial fat loss and fat descent

A youthful face is padded with facial fat in the right places, has full features in the mid and upper face. This makes a typical youthful face somewhat triangular in shape. The fat in the face is divided into various compartments, and in particular fat compartments within the cheek are vital to full, prominent cheeks.

The fat cells in the subcutaneous layer get smaller with age. Age-related facial fat atrophy leads to a sunken appearance in cheeks, temples and eye sockets.

The cheek paddings do not only thin out; they also descend, resulting in flattening cheeks, the appearance of prominent nose-to-mouth folds, a groove under the eye and the jawline becoming less distinct. As the fat compartments of the cheeks migrate into a lower position, the whole face becomes more squarish in shape.

Facial bone thinning

Previous studies have found that facial bones lose volume with age. The degree of age-related facial bone changes varies considerably from person to person. Women show the changes earlier than men since women tend to lose bone tissue faster because of menopause-related changes. For example, the cheekbones become less prominent and the lower jaw shrinks.

Thinning facial bones are less able to support the overlying soft tissues – muscles, fat and skin. That results in facial sagging and drooping. Any shortening of teeth may further increase the signs of ageing in the area around the lips and mouth.

Facial muscle atrophy

With age the facial muscles tend to reduce in size, strength and tone in a similar way to other skeletal muscles of the body. Muscle mass is lost because both the number and size of muscle fibres decrease. As facial muscles loosen and atrophy, this contributes to facial volume loss, sagging, droopiness and an aged look.

It is important to note that the changes are more the result of inactivity than the direct result of age. The body works on the principle of 'use it or lose it' and muscle atrophy is caused by not using the muscles enough.

In most people the facial muscles are not well understood and they are not controlled consciously. The reason why facial muscles gradually atrophy is because they are seldom asked to perform effectively varied movements in the full range of motion available to them.

Facial fascia and ligament weakening

Facial muscles are connected to the dermis by one continuous organized fibrous network, called SMAS (superficial musculoaponeurotic system). The retaining ligaments anchor the facial soft tissues to the underlying facial bones. With ageing, the retaining ligaments weaken and are less able to hold up the skin and fat compartments. Fascial, ligamentous and muscular weakening and laxity result in the sagging of all the elements of soft tissues.

FACIAL SAGGING

- eyebrows descend
- eyebags
- upper cheeks flatten
- nasolabial folds
- sagging jawline
- jowls
- drooping nasal tip

FACIAL **LINES**

Facial lines and creases can exist in an otherwise wrinkle-free face. Facial lines result from tightened mimic muscles. These lines travel crosswise to the muscle cells in the mimic muscles. Fine lines turn into deep creases and furrows when skin in the bottom of the facial line becomes thinner and the connective collagen network of the skin deteriorates.

Temporary and permanent facial lines

Mimic muscles differ from other muscles of the body by attaching partly to the skin. When the mimic muscle contracts, it causes the overlying skin to move.

For example, contraction of the frontalis muscle raises the eyebrows and creates horizontal lines and folds on the forehead. This happens to people of all ages. When eyebrows lower and the frontalis muscle relaxes, the lines and folds on the forehead smooth, especially at a young age.

Certain habitual facial expressions tighten and shorten the mimic muscles. Taut and shortened mimic muscles pull the skin covering it into pleats, and over the years facial lines become gradually permanent. Even people under the age of 30 may have creases created like this.

1   Horizontal forehead creases appear when the frontalis muscle tightens.

2   Vertical glabellar furrows, or 'frown lines', result from tightening of the corrugator supercilii muscle and depressor supercilii muscle.

3   Transverse creases at the nasal bridge are caused by tightening of the procerus muscle.

4   Lines around the eyes, or 'crows feet', are formed when the orbicularis oculi muscle tightens.

5   Vertical lip lines, or perioral rhytides or 'smoker's lines' are induced by tightening of superficial muscle fibres of the orbicularis oris muscle.

6   Nose-to-mouth lines, or nasolabial lines, result from tightening of the muscles which elevate the corner of the mouth and the upper lip.

7   Lines going down from the corners of the mouth, or 'marionette lines', are formed when the depressor anguli oris muscle tightens.

8   Horizontal mental or chin crease is caused by tightening of the mentalis muscle.

9   Horizontal creases and vertical bands on the neck result from tightening of the platysma muscle.

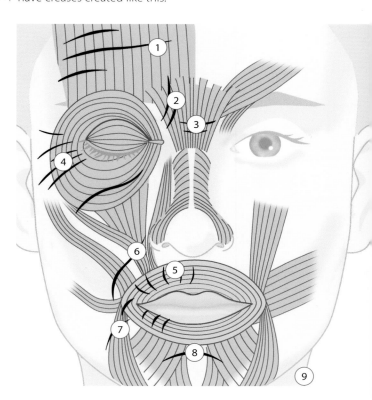

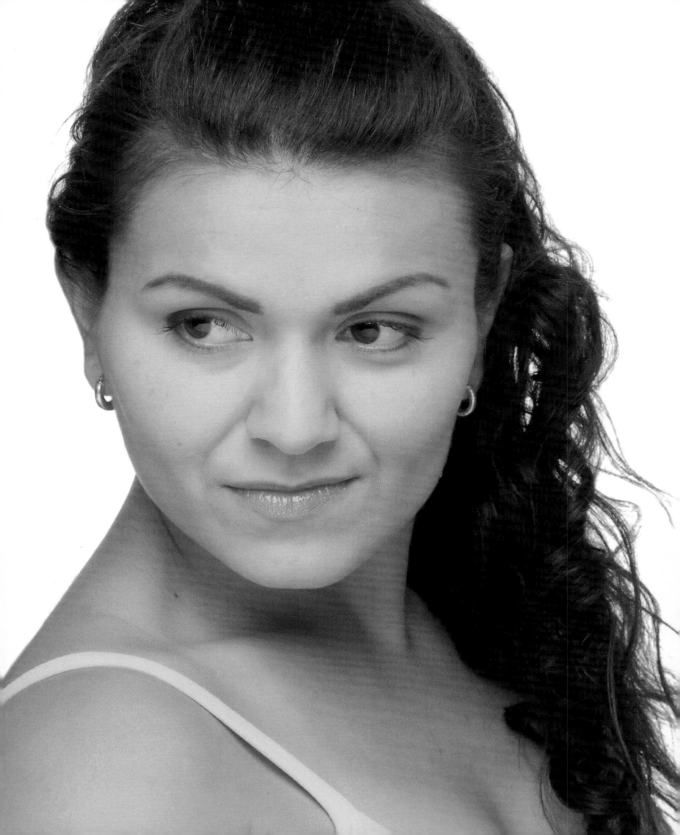

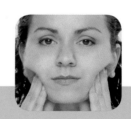

MUSCLES AND
MUSCLE TENSION OF
THE FACIAL AREA

4

MUSCLES OF **THE FACIAL REGION**

The muscles of the facial area are the mimic muscles and the chewing muscles. The movements of the mimic muscles create facial expressions and the chewing muscles move the lower jawbone. The structure of these muscles corresponds to that of other muscles in the body responsible for initiating motion.

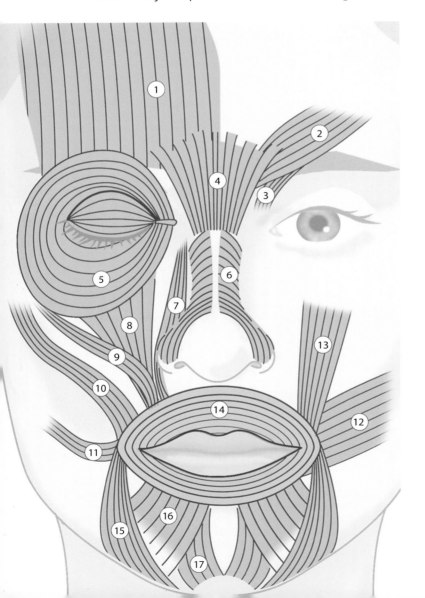

MIMIC MUSCLES

1   Frontalis muscle

2   Corrugator supercilii muscle

3   Depressor supercilii muscle

4   Procerus muscle

5   Orbicularis oculi muscle

6   Nasalis muscle

7   Levator labii superioris alaeque nasi muscle

8   Levator labii superioris muscle

9   Zygomaticus minor muscle

10   Zygomaticus major muscle

11   Risorius muscle

12   Buccinator muscle

13   Levator anguli oris muscle

14   Orbicularis oris muscle

15   Depressor anguli oris muscle

16   Depressor labii inferioris muscle

17   Mentalis muscle

The superficial layer of the mimic muscles is shown on one side of the face, and the deep layer on the other half (muscles 2, 3,12,13).

Mimic muscles create facial expressions

Muscles in the torso and limbs travel over joints. They are connected to bones and are responsible for putting the body in motion. Facial muscles do not play a role as joint movers. Facial muscles are only partly attached to the facial bones and primarily to the skin of the face.

When mimic muscles contract, they cause the overlying skin to move and the face to make expressions. In addition to creating expressions, facial muscles are employed when talking, eating and drinking.

Mimic muscles are arranged around eyes, mouth and nose. Most mimic muscles come in pairs, one on each side of the face. Motor cells of the facial nerve send signals to the mimic muscles to move.

Chewing muscles move the lower jawbone

Chewing muscles (masticatory muscles) work as joint movers, because they move the lower jawbone, which articulates with the skull at the jaw joints. There are four pairs of chewing muscles and they are arranged around the jaw joints.

Chewing muscles are stronger than mimic muscles, because biting needs much more muscle strength than, for example, raising the eyebrows. Chewing muscles can press something between the back teeth with the force of around 70 kilograms.

Chewing muscles are used for chewing food and moving the lower jawbone while speaking. Motor cells of the trigeminal nerve send signals to the chewing muscles to move.

CHEWING MUSCLES

1 Temporalis muscle
2 Masseter muscle, superficial part
3 Masseter muscle, deep part
4 Medial pterygoid muscle
5 Lateral pterygoid muscle

MIMIC MUSCLES

The mimic muscles are arranged in pairs around the eye, the mouth and the nose. Mimic muscles move the skin of the face and create expressions. They are also active during speaking and eating and serve a protective function for the eyes. Some individual differences exist in the attachments of the mimic muscles as well in their size and development.

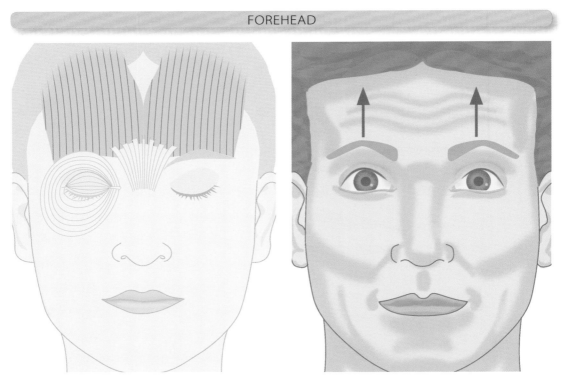

FOREHEAD

Frontalis muscle (forehead muscle) is part of the occipitofrontalis muscle, which begins at the back of the head and ends at the eyebrows. The frontalis muscle raises the eyebrows and the skin between the eyebrows. The contraction of the frontalis muscle creates horizontal skinfolds and lines on the forehead. Because the frontalis muscle is a paired muscle, it is possible to raise each eyebrow separately.

AREA BETWEEN THE EYEBROWS

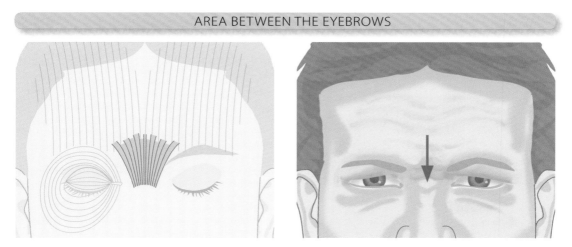

A) Corrugator supercilii muscle (frowning muscle) pulls the eyebrows together and makes vertical skinfolds and lines between the eyebrows. It lies deep to the procerus and frontalis muscles.

B) Depressor supercilii muscle works with the corrugator supercilii muscle, pulling the eyebrows together downwards. It is located just below corrugator muscle.

AREA BETWEEN THE EYEBROWS

Procerus muscle draws downwards the medial corners of eyebrows and the skin between the eyebrows, thus producing horizontal skinfolds and lines into the base of nose.

EYE

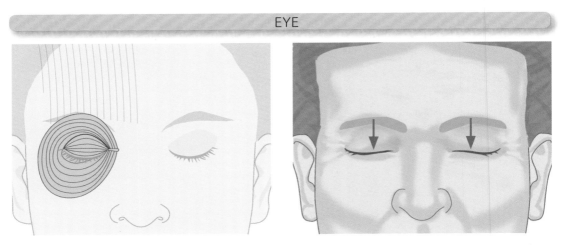

Orbicularis oculi muscle forms a broad ring-like muscular layer around the eyes, spreading downwards on the cheeks. The area of the muscle that occupies the eyelids is called the palpebral portion. The area covering the entire eye socket is known as the orbital portion.

The orbicularis oculi muscle closes the eyes and spreads tears over the cornea. The palpebral portion closes the eyelids gently, but when more force is required, when closing the eyes tightly and squinting, the orbital portion is also engaged. Contraction of the orbicularis oculi muscle causes lines around the eyes.

CHEEKBONE

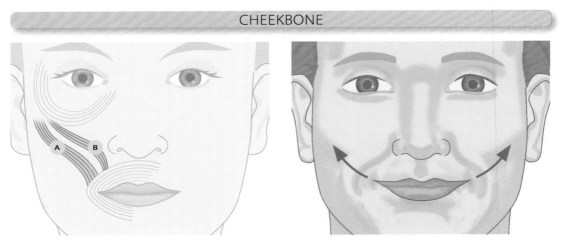

A) Zygomaticus major muscle
B) Zygomaticus minor muscle
These muscles receive their names from the bone they are attached to, the zygomatic bone (cheekbone), and are used for smiling and laughing. Zygomaticus major runs into the corner of the mouth and zygomaticus minor into the upper lip. Zygomaticus major is longer and thicker than zygomaticus minor.

CHEEK

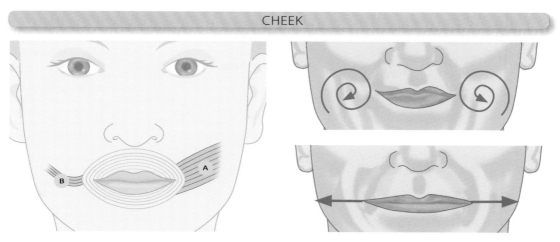

A) **Buccinator muscle** is situated deep and makes up the interior wall of the cheek. The buccinator muscle pulls the corners of the mouth sideways and compresses the cheeks so that during chewing food is pushed beneath the molar teeth. The buccinator muscle is also employed in whistling or blowing, as well as playing the trumpet, hence its name 'the trumpet muscle'.

B) **Risorius muscle** pulls the corners of the mouth sideways and makes a grinning facial expression. The risorius muscle can produce dimples in some individuals.

MOUTH

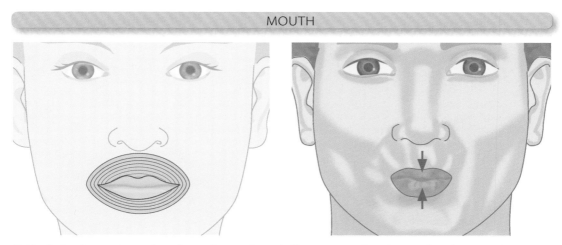

Orbicularis oris muscle consists of many layers of muscle fibres surrounding the mouth and creates the basic structure of the lips. Many of its fibres are connected with the fibres of other facial muscles such as the buccinator muscle and the other muscles at the corner of the mouth. This complex arrangement makes possible the varied movements of the lips such as closing or pressing the lips together, protruding them forward in a 'kissing' action and all the precise changes of the shape of the mouth needed in pronunciation.

MIDFACE

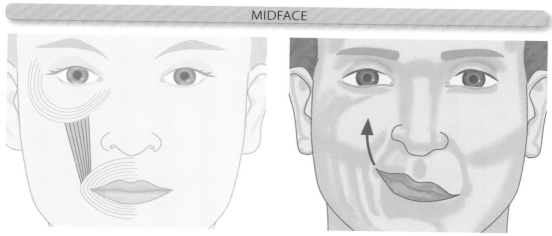

Levator anguli oris muscle is inserted into the corner of the mouth and pulls it upward.
It is positioned beneath the levator labii superioris and zygomaticus major muscles.

MIDFACE

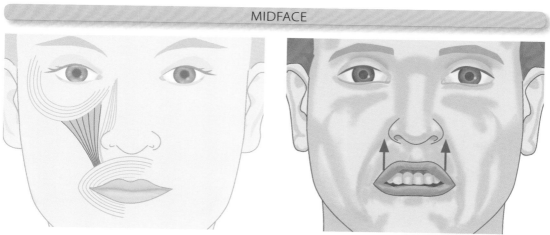

Levator labii superioris muscle is inserted into the skin of the upper lip.
It elevates the upper lip and rolls the upper lip outward.

MIDFACE

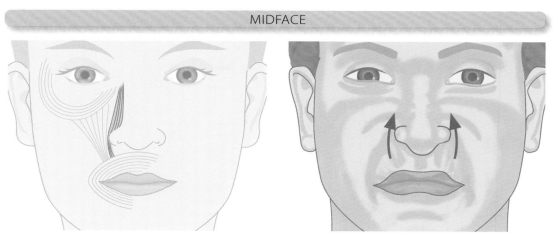

Levator labii superioris alaeque nasi muscle is attached to the upper lip and to the lateral part of the nostrils. It elevates the upper lip and aids in dilation of the nostrils.

CHIN

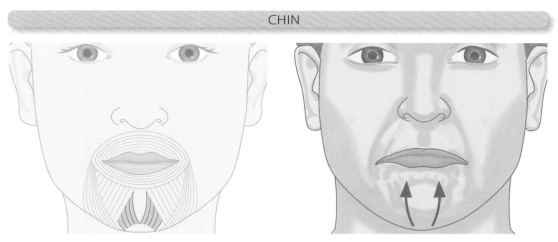

Mentalis muscle (chin muscle) is inserted into the skin on the chin. When contracting, it pulls the skin of the chin upwards, causes a transverse line in the chin and wrinkles the skin of the chin – for instance, when a person is about to cry.

CHIN

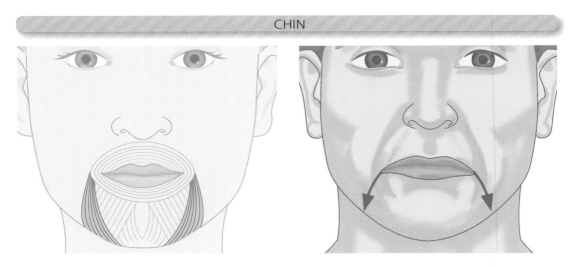

Depressor anguli oris muscle is a triangular-shaped muscle. It is inserted into the corner of the mouth and draws it downward. Contraction of the depressor anguli oris muscle over time results in 'marionette lines'.

CHIN

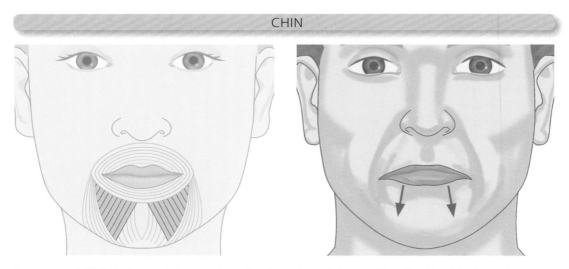

Depressor labii inferioris muscle is a quadrangular-shaped muscle inserted into the skin of the lower lip. It depresses the lower lip and protrudes it, as in pouting.

NECK

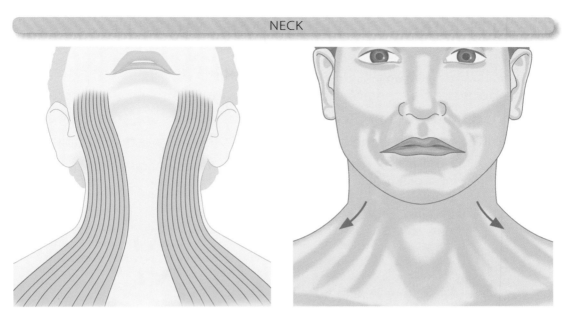

Platysma muscle is a flat, broad and very thin muscle sheet extending from the lower face over the collar bones on to the chest area. Even though the platysma muscle is situated mainly in front of the neck, it belongs to the mimic muscles, because it is partly attached to the skin, creates facial expressions and is innervated by the facial nerve. The platysma muscle draws the corner of mouth downward, tenses the skin of the neck and assists in depressing the lower jawbone.

NOSE   EAR

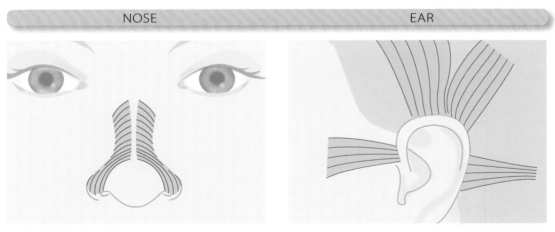

Nasalis muscle has a transverse part that narrows the nostrils and a smaller alar part that widens the nostrils.

Three muscles connect the ear with the scalp, but these muscles are not important for human facial expressions.

TIGHTENING OF THE MIMIC MUSCLES

Facial muscles become tensed and tight just like other muscles of the body. Facial tension affects both your health and appearance. Prolonged unfavourable, usually unconscious habitual expressions can lead to headache and facial pain and will in time be seen in permanent facial lines, reflecting these individual facial habits.

Tensed muscle of the forehead

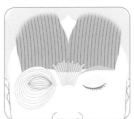

CAUSES OF TENSION: The function of the forehead's muscle, the frontalis muscle, is to draw the eyebrows and the skin of the forehead upwards. Excessive raising of the eyebrows is a common, mostly unconscious facial habit. Many people raise their eyebrows when they talk and when they sing. Some older individuals simply need to raise their eyebrows to open their eyes in order to see better. The reason for this is excess lax skin of the upper eyelid or drooping eyebrow which causes the skin of the upper lid to bunch. Eyebrows must be raised to counteract these changes.

IMPACT ON APPEARANCE: Chronic contraction of the frontalis muscle affects facial appearance by creating gradually permanent horizontal creases running across in the skin of the forehead.

IMPACT ON HEALTH: A tensed and tight frontalis muscle can affect your health by causing local pain over the forehead. If a tight frontalis muscle traps the supraorbital nerve (a sensory branch of the trigeminal nerve) the consequence is a migraine-like headache.

The frontalis is the front part of the occipito-frontalis muscle which covers the head from the back of the head to the forehead. The back part is called the occipitalis muscle. The frontalis and occipitalis act together, retracting the skin of the forehead even further, opening the eyes more widely. The pain from the tensed occipitalis muscle spreads from the back of the head through the top of the head, and can cause intense pain behind the eye (deep in the eye socket. Those experiencing deep, aching pain due to a tensed occipitalis may find that putting the weight of the back of their head on the pillow will increase the ache and thus prefer lying on their side.

Tensed muscles between the eyebrows

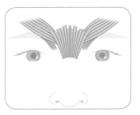

CAUSES OF TENSION: The muscles between the eyebrows, including the corrugator supercilii, procerus and depressor supercilii muscles, draw the eyebrows together and down as in frowning. People draw their eyebrows downwards and towards the middle to protect their eyes from bright sunlight. Some people frown frequently when they concentrate and some people have a habit of frowning a lot when they talk.

IMPACT ON APPEARANCE: The muscles mainly responsible for frowning are the corrugator and depressor supercilii muscles. A distinctive facial habit of frowning will in time tighten these muscles and lead to formation of permanent vertical glabellar furrows. A deep horizontal line over the bridge of the nose is the result of chronic contraction of the procerus. The procerus muscle often contracts in activities requiring some effort.

IMPACT ON HEALTH: Tensed and tight corrugaror/depressor supercilii complex can compress a nerve penetrating them. The compressed nerve is a small sensory branch of the trigeminal nerve, called the supratrochlear nerve. When this nerve is irritated, it can induce a migraine-like headache.

Tensed muscles around the eyes

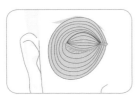

CAUSES OF TENSION: Habitual squinting for any reason tenses the ring muscle of the eye, the orbicularis oculi muscle. Sunlight causes us to squint. Nearsighted people not wearing glasses squint to improve their vision to see objects in the distance more clearly.

IMPACT ON APPEARANCE: Chronic tension of orbicularis oculi creates and deepens lines around the eyes. Tight orbicularis oculi also pulls the outer part of the eyebrow down, resulting in descending of the outer edge of the eyebrow.

IMPACT ON HEALTH: Tensed orbicularis oculi muscle may cause local pain above the upper eyelid just below the eyebrow. Some individuals with a tensed and tight orbicularis oculi muscle may have a reading problem where strong black letters on white background seem to jump, making it difficult to focus on them.

Tensed muscles around the mouth

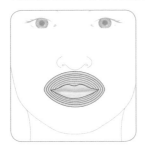

CAUSES OF TENSION: The ring muscle around the mouth, the orbicularis oris muscle, closes the lips. The habit of pursing the lips excessively and pressing the lips tightly together tenses and tightens the orbicularis oris.

IMPACT ON APPEARANCE: Tightening of the orbicularis oris will in time lead to lines and creases around the lips. A tightened orbicularis oris also makes the lips look thinner.

IMPACT ON HEALTH: Tension and tightness of the orbicularis oris and other mimic muscles attaching to orbicularis oris muscle have a negative effect on speaking by creating unnecessary tension in these mimic muscles needed in pronunciation.

Tensed mimic muscles below the mouth

CAUSES OF TENSION: An unfavourable facial habit of turning the corners of the mouth downward will tighten the muscles below the mouth.

IMPACT ON APPEARANCE: Because of the tightening of the depressor anguli oris and platysma muscles, the corners of the mouth are eventually permanently turned downwards with lines running down to the chin, known as marionette lines. In old age the tight platysma muscle is the producer of horizontal neck creases and platysmal bands.

Other tensed mimic muscles

IMPACT ON HEALTH: Problems of the chewing muscles can irritate nearby muscles such as the buccinator and zygomaticus major muscles. Tensed buccinator muscle may cause local pain deep in the cheek. Tensed zygomaticus major refers pain along the side of the nose up to the middle of the forehead.

TENSED FACIAL MUSCULATURE

When the facial musculature is chronically tensed and contracted, the face looks tired and stressed out, feels stiff and tight, and a headache is a common symptom.

CHEWING MUSCLES

The primary function of the chewing muscles (muscles of mastication) is to raise the lower jawbone and thus to close the mouth. They also draw the lower jaw forward and back, move it from side to side and in a circular motion. Precise and delicate work of these muscles of chewing and biting is necessary for eating and vital for speech production.

TEMPLE AREA

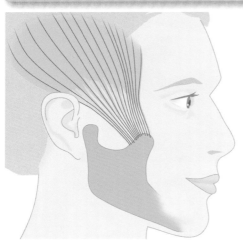

Temporalis muscle is a broad, fan-shaped muscle which covers the temple area. It originates from the side of the skull, passes under the zygomatic arch and its fibres converge into a tendon that inserts into the lower jawbone. The temporalis muscle is one of the three chewing muscles that closes the jaw.

The posterior fibres of the temporalis muscle are important for drawing the lower jawbone back and sideways. Temporalis is capable of coordinating jaw-closing movements and thus it is an important muscle in maintaining the resting position of the lower jaw.

CHEEK AREA

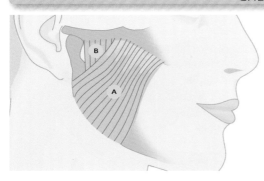

Masseter muscle is a square-shaped jaw-closer, which acts in conjunction with the temporalis. It is a thick and powerful muscle that brings the teeth together and provides the force necessary to chew and bite efficiently.

The masseter muscle is in two layers, superficial (A) and deep (B). Both parts run from the zygomatic arch to the angle of the lower jawbone.

BEHIND THE JAWBONE

Medial pterygoid and lateral pterygoid muscles are two different jaw muscles. They are situated deep in the jaw and both are named according to their common attachment to the skull region called the pterygoid process.

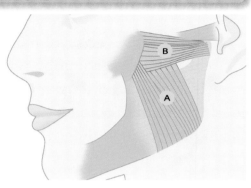

A) Medial pterygoid muscle is the third jaw-closer and works as a synergistic partner with the masseter muscle to aid in elevating the lower jaw. Besides raising the lower jaw, the medial pterygoid muscle protrudes it and pulls it sideways.

Medial pterygoid lies in the deeper plane and is hidden by the back of the lower jawbone. The medial pterygoid muscle on the inside of the jawbone and the masseter muscle on the outside form a musclular sling that supports the lower jaw at the jaw angle.

B) Lateral pterygoid muscle is situated deep to the zygomatic arch and is divided into two anatomically separate short muscles. The smaller, upper part has attachments to the jaw joint capsule and the disc within it. The lower part has attachments to the head of the lower jawbone.

The lateral pterygoid muscle is involved in lowering the jaw by protruding the lower jaw and moving the articular disc forward. It is also active during the side-to-side movements of the jaw, as in chewing and grinding.

UNDER THE JAWBONE

Digastric muscle is not generally classified as one of the muscles of the mastication, although its important function is to open the jaw. The digastric muscle originates from the skull, passes through a fibrous loop attached to the hyoid bone, and then inserts to the undersurface of the lower jawbone. The hyoid bone is a small, U-shaped bone located between the lower jawbone and the Adam's apple (the larynx).

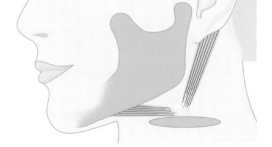

Other muscles influencing the lower jaw

The jaw-closing muscles are much stronger than the jaw-opening muscles. Besides the digastric and lateral pterygoid muscles, the jaw is lowered by the force of gravity and by a group of muscles running between the lower jawbone and the lingual bone (hyoid bone), called the suprahyoid muscles.

The lingual bone is connected to the breast bone, collar bones and shoulder blades by the infrahyoid muscles. Together with the suprahyoid muscles, they can support the lingual bone, providing a firm base on which the lower jawbone can be moved.

Muscles moving the head, such as sternoclei-domastoid muscle and the muscles at the back of the neck that are attached to the skull, play a big part in positioning the head.

Head posture affects the position of the lower jawbone. For example, a forward head posture may cause a harmful change in the position of the lower jaw and strain the chewing muscles.

TIGHTENING OF THE CHEWING MUSCLES

An unhealthy, mostly unconscious habit of clenching and grinding the teeth is a common reason behind tight and tensed chewing muscles. Increased tension of the chewing muscles can eventually lead to health problems such as a stiff jaw, sore temples, headache, facial pain, pain in the jaw joint and ringing in the ears.

Bad daytime habits

Clenching of the jaw is a natural and common reaction in response to many aspects of daily living. Many people clench their teeth when they are concentrating on a task such as driving a car or working at a computer. If you are feeling annoyed and irritated and need to repress these feelings, if you are feeling impatient when stuck in a traffic jam or feeling anxious when having a busy schedule, it is common to clench the jaw, tighten the jaw muscles, 'grit one's teeth'. It is also common to press the teeth together during strenuous physical activities such as lifting weights.

The habit of clenching the teeth too much and too often is an unhealthy, harmful habit with regard to the muscles and joints. Some people clench their teeth a lot, often being unaware of this action. If one habitually clenches one's jaw, it strains the chewing muscles and the jaw joints, eventually resulting in pains and dysfunction of the muscles and joints.

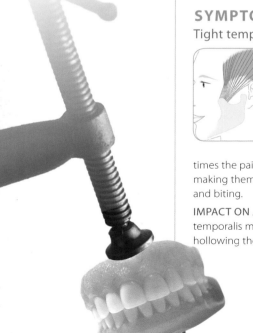

SYMPTOMS OF TIGHT CHEWING MUSCLES

Tight temporalis muscle

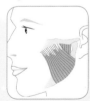

IMPACT ON HEALTH: Headache is a common symptom caused by the tensed temporalis muscle. The pain is felt widely over the temples, along the eyebrows and behind the eye. Sometimes the pain refers to the upper teeth, making them hypersensitive to cold, heat and biting.

IMPACT ON APPEARANCE: Tensed and tight temporalis muscle affects the appearance by hollowing the temples.

Tight masseter muscle

IMPACT ON HEALTH: Tightness of the masseter muscle limits the opening of the jaw. The lower jaw feels stiff and fatigues easily. A tensed and tight masseter muscle causes pain in the area of the muscle itself and refers pain to the lower and upper jaw, above the eyebrows, to the region of the jaw joint and deep into the ear. Referred pain to the back teeth makes them hypersensitive to pressure and temperature changes. A tensed and tight masseter muscle can also cause tinnitus.

IMPACT ON APPEARANCE: A tight masseter muscle affects the appearance by decreasing the healthy and youthful fullness and roundness of the cheeks.

Even worse night-time activities

A small amount of chewing muscle activity during the sleep is quite normal, but waking up in the morning with a stiff jaw or a headache spreading over the temples may reveal an excessive clenching or grinding of one's teeth when asleep.

Sleep studies have discovered that the group of nocturnal teeths clenchers and grinders spent about 40 minutes with their teeth together during eight hours of sleep, whereas the control group kept their teeth together for only about five minutes. Clenching and grinding events were associated with a change from deeper to lighter sleep. External disturbances, such as sounds, touch and flashing lights, have been shown to induce the sleeper's teeth grinding.

Clenching the teeth occurs both in the daytime and in night-time, but it is typically much more forceful during the sleep. The clenching power of the nocturnal clenchers was significantly high, often exceeding the force of normal chewing.

Grinding the teeth together is mainly a night-time activity. The sound of grinding the teeth can be so loud and disruptive that another person in the same room hears it easily. Nocturnal teeth clenching and especially teeth grinding do not only stress the jaw musculature and joints but also destroy the tooth enamel.

Unbalanced bite

In addition to moving the lower jawbone while talking and eating, a slight activity of the chewing muscles keeps the lower jaw closed in the right resting position. When the upper and lower teeth have the right height and meet in harmony, the bite is correct and the chewing muscles are able to find a suitable resting place for the lower jawbone with minimum effort.

Changes in bite (occlusion), especially with a decreased vertical dimension due to worn, flattened teeth or other changes due to missing back (molar) teeth, dental fillings that are too high, poorly fitting crowns, implants or dentures can lead to an unbalanced bite. It becomes harder for the chewing muscles to find a proper resting position for the lower jaw and the tension increases in the overworking chewing muscles.

Tight medial pterygoid muscle

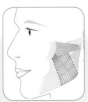

IMPACT ON HEALTH: A feeling of stuffiness and pressure in the ear may be a symptom of a tight medial pterygoid muscle. This happens when a tight medial pterygoid disturbs the opening action of the eustachian tube, the canal connecting the middle ear to the throat. The medial pterygoid refers pain below and behind the jaw joint and deep in the ear.

Tight lateral pterygoid muscle

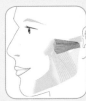

IMPACT ON HEALTH: The lateral pterygoid muscle has attachments to the disc within the jaw joint and tightness of the muscle disturbs the movements of the disc. Clicking sounds in the jaw joint may result from the tight lateral pterygoid muscle. A tensed and tight lateral pterygoid muscle causes pain in the jaw joint. The referred pain in the upper jaw may feel the same as the pain of a sinus attack (sinusitis).

Tight digastric muscle

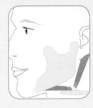

IMPACT ON HEALTH: The digastric muscle is located below the lower jaw and assists in opening the jaw against the counterforce of the powerful jaw-closing chewing muscles. Overload due to teeth clenching and grinding tenses end tightens the digastric muscle. As the digastiric muscle has attachments to the hyoid bone, the symptoms may be a difficulty in swallowing, a feeling of a lump in the throat.

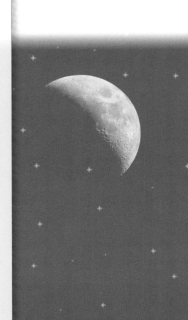

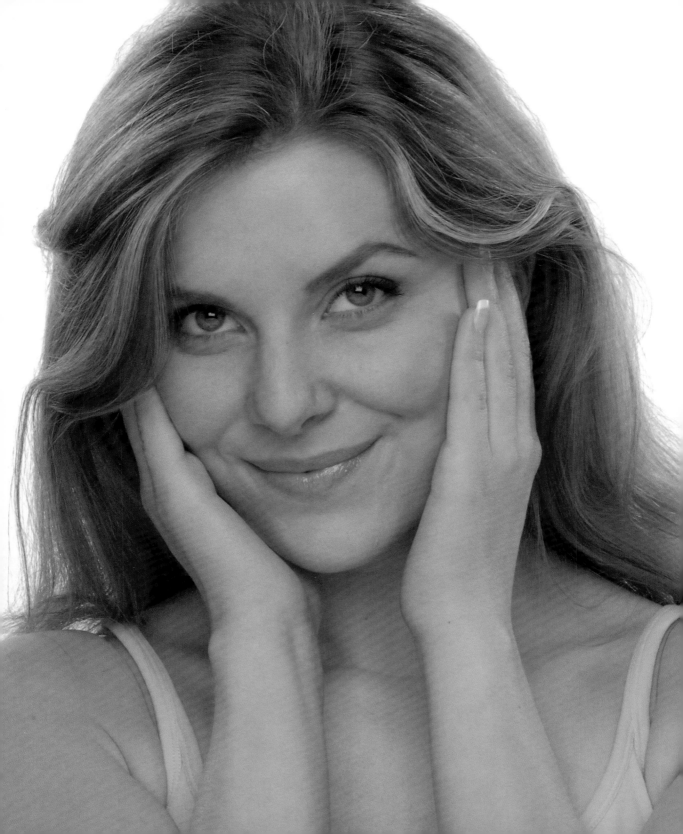

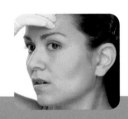

HOW TO TAKE CARE OF
THE MUSCLES OF
THE FACIAL AREA
5

GENERAL INSTRUCTIONS

MimiLift techniques will improve both your health and facial appearance. The impacts of the procedures are clearly explained, so you can choose the right programme for your individual situation, needs and goals.

Awareness and knowledge

Where there is muscular weakness or incoordination, strengthening and movement exercises are needed. Appropriate MimiLift exercises correct and prevent atrophy, weakness and functional impairment of the facial musculature.

MimiLift Facial MuscleCare will develop your awareness of your face, of your facial habits and your ability to differentiate parts of your facial area that are tense. You will learn to discover where you are tensing inappropriate muscles or where you are making an effort when none is necessary. Through regular practice you will be familiar with the feeling of a relaxed face and jaw.

Relaxed does not mean flaccid. Relaxation is an activity, the ability to eliminate unnecessary tension. True relaxation improves your health and vitality. The more you become aware of the difference between tension and relaxation and the contrast between how you feel before and after practice, the easier you can change the old, tensing habits, and you will be able to achieve results with shorter and shorter practice sessions.

INSTRUCTIONS

- You do not have to perform all the MimiLift procedures instructed in this book. Their effects are explained in order to help you to develop an individual programme for yourself. You choose the best procedures for your personal needs.

- Muscle-based facial pains and headaches are correctable conditions, not a disease. You can relieve the pain by gently massaging and stretching the tensed and tight muscles. However, do not treat only the symptoms. Try to find the reasons behind them, and try to eliminate the sources of the problem.

- Do not hurry through all the procedures at once. First of all read the instructions and the theory parts of the book carefully. Learn to understand the anatomy and physiology of your face. Choosing the right exercises and performing them correctly is important.

- Start with only a few procedures and perform them for few days. Then add some new procedures. Give yourself time to learn each procedure. Listen to your face and jaw. Some of the procedures might feel a little strange or cause some discomfort in the beginning, but none of the exercises should elicit pain.

- Perform the procedures at first 4–6 times a week, once or twice a day. MimiLift procedures can be done whenever and wherever – for example, when watching TV. After a few weeks, having achieved results, you can maintain the results by performing the procedures 2–4 times a week. If you have a few days' or a couple of weeks' break, the results won't disappear.

- You will feel the impact of MimiLift procedures on your muscle tone and on your facial circulation even immediately. More evident results can be expected after a few weeks of regular and committed practice.

  CAUTION: Thin, hygienic, well-fitting, medical-grade gloves are recommended, especially when placing the fingers inside the mouth. Make sure that the gloves do not contain material that might cause allergic reactions.

MOVEMENT EXERCISES FOR THE JAW

The jaw exercises of MimiLift Facial MuscleCare improve the endurance, strength and elasticity of the chewing muscles. Well-conditioned and well-functioning chewing muscles are important in creating normal, healthy movements of the jaw.

Benefits

Rhythmic, smooth jaw movements encourage ideal function of the chewing muscles and jaw joints and help to restore optimal range of movements of the jaw. They also reduce stiffness and pain of the chewing muscles and jaw joints.

Resisted jaw exercises strengthen the chewing muscles and ligaments that support the jaw joints. In addition to strengthening effects, resistance exercises create a reflex muscle reaction, which relaxes the chewing muscles.

Jaw exercises train all the muscles operating the jaw to work in harmony with each other and on each side and help the jaw joints and disc movements to function in precise synchronized harmony. Jaw exercises also produce normal and necessary functional loading to the articular surfaces of the jaw joints. These tissues need a certain amount of loading to stay healthy because loading forces drive synovial fluid in and out of the articular surfaces, bringing nutrients and carrying waste products away.

INSTRUCTIONS

- Perform all the jaw exercises slowly, carefully, smoothly and evenly.

- Concentrate on creating controlled, well-coordinated and fluent jaw movements.

- Maintain a good upper body posture with the head well-aligned when doing the jaw exercises.

- Focus on your jaw and your neck. Carry the jaw exercises in a relaxed manner. Keep your neck and shoulders relaxed.

- When performing manual resistance jaw exercises, apply just a gentle and light resistance with your fingers.

- Repeat each exercise the recommended number of times. You can increase the number of repetitions if you like.

- All the jaw exercises should be painless. They might feel a little strange or cause some discomfort at the beginning, but if any exercise produces pain, decrease the force or the range of movement or both. If a certain jaw movement still elicits pain, do not continue performing it, because pain may be a symptom of a jaw joint problem needing further medical evaluation.

CAUTION: Never apply maximum resistance or perform sudden, forceful jaw movements or try to force your jaw to make movements that exceed the normal range of motion of the jaw joints. Those with a history of a jaw dislocation must be careful not to perform movements of the jaw that are too wide.

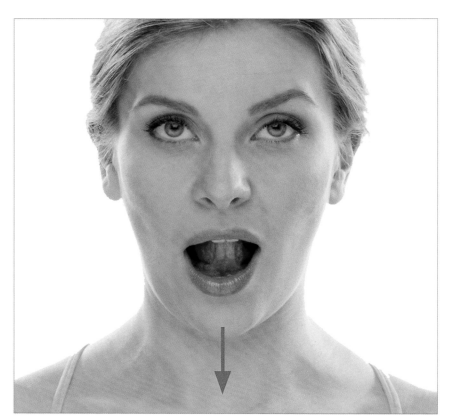

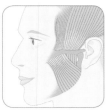

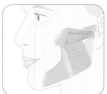

1 Coordinated jaw opening exercise

Place the tip of your tongue against the roof of your mouth behind the front teeth and open your jaw slowly. Lower your jaw as far as you can while keeping your tongue tip up. Hold your jaw in this position for 2 seconds.

Alternate opening and closing your jaw slowly while keeping your tongue tip up. Repeat 10 times.

IMPACT ON HEALTH: Helps the straight, smooth downward direction of the lower jaw without any deviations during the movement.

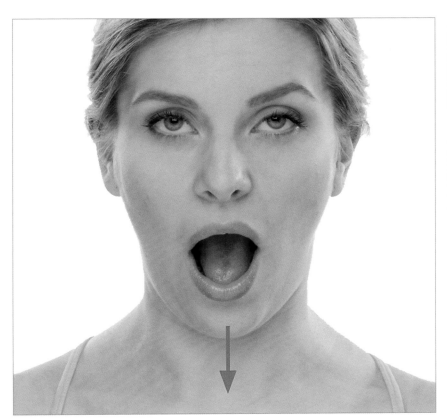
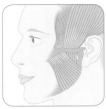
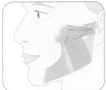

2 Basic jaw opening exercise

Open your mouth by lowering your jaw slowly and evenly as wide as feels comfortable. Hold in the open position for 2 seconds. Alternate opening and closing your jaw slowly and smoothly. Repeat 10 times.

Concentrate on the straight downward direction of the lower jaw without deviations or clicking sounds during the movement. If there is a click, it is usually eliminated by bringing the lower jaw slightly forward and then open.

IMPACT ON HEALTH: Improves the function and condition of the chewing muscles and jaw joints. Relaxes jaw-closing chewing muscles. Helps speech and swallowing.

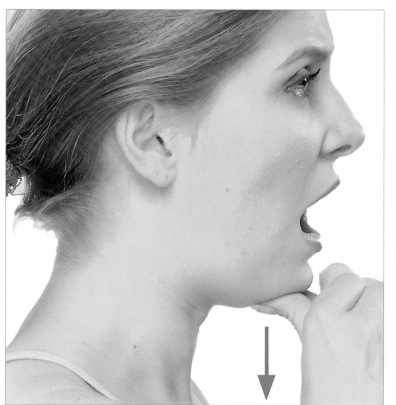

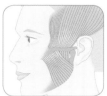

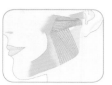

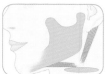

3 Resisted jaw opening exercise

Place your thumbs firmly underneath the tip of your chin. Open your jaw slowly and resist the opening slightly and gently with your thumbs. The resistance subtly resists the active movement without stopping it.

Gradually decrease the amount of resistance applied as your lower jaw approaches the furthest open position. Slowly release the resistance and return your lower jaw to the resting position. Repeat 10 times.

IMPACT ON HEALTH: Relaxes jaw-closing chewing muscles. Strengthens jaw-opening muscles.

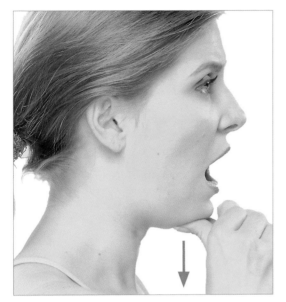
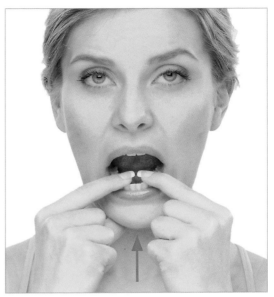

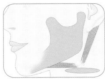
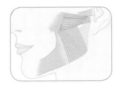
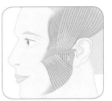

4 Combined jaw-opening and jaw-closing exercise with resistance

At first place your thumbs firmly underneath the tip of your chin. Open your jaw and resist the opening with your thumbs. Then place your index fingers over your front lower teeth and gently resist the jaw-closing movement. Repeat 10 times.

The resistance subtly resists the active movements without stopping them. The movements should be slow and even and the resistance gentle.

> **IMPACT ON HEALTH:** Strengthens the chewing muscles and jaw joints. Relaxes jaw-closing chewing muscles.
> **IMPACT ON APPEARANCE:** Tones the cheeks.

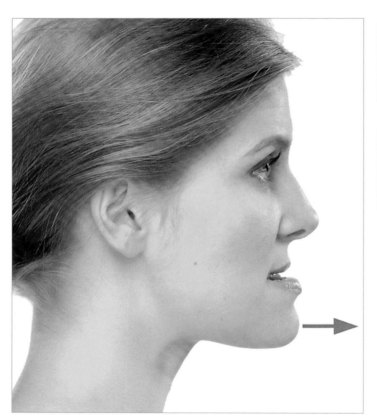
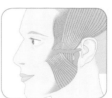
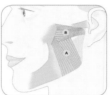

5 Basic jaw forward thrust exercise

Move your lower jaw slightly forward. Hold your jaw in this position for 3–5 seconds. Return your jaw slowly to the resting position. Repeat 10 times. Focus on moving your lower jaw without moving your neck.

Average normal jaw protrusion movement varies between 7 mm and 12 mm.

IMPACT ON HEALTH: Relaxes and stretches jaw-retracting chewing muscles. Corrects muscle-based incorrect bite, in which the lower jaw has gone back too far.

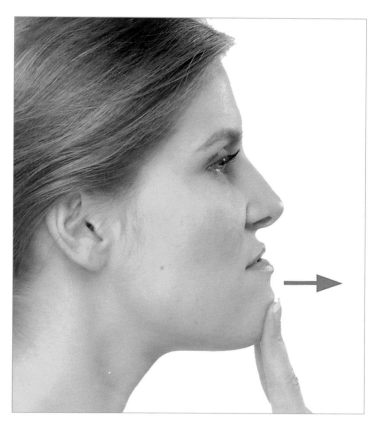

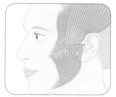

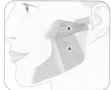

6 Resisted jaw forward thrust exercise

Place the index and middle fingers of your both hands against your chin. Move your lower jaw slightly forward and resist the movement lightly and gently with your fingers. The resistance subtly resists the active movement without stopping it. Repeat 10 times.

IMPACT ON HEALTH: Relaxes and stretches jaw-retracting chewing muscles. Strengthens jaw-protruding chewing muscles. Promotes the natural pathway of the jaw-opening motion.

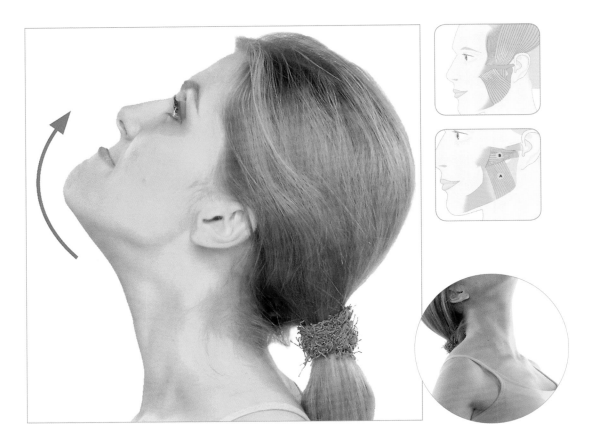

7 Jaw forward thrust exercise with front neck stretch

Move your lower jaw forward and then upwards so that you can extend your lower lip widely over your upper lip. Keep your jaw and lips like this and tilt your head slightly back. The tip of your tongue is placed against the roof of your mouth and your chest is lifted.

Hold this position for 3–5 seconds. You will feel a stretch around the jawline and in the front of your neck. Return your head and jaw slowly to the neutral position. Repeat 5 times.

IMPACT ON HEALTH: Relaxes and stretches jaw-retracting chewing muscles and the front neck muscles.
IMPACT ON APPEARANCE: Tones the jawline. Prevents and softens neck creases.

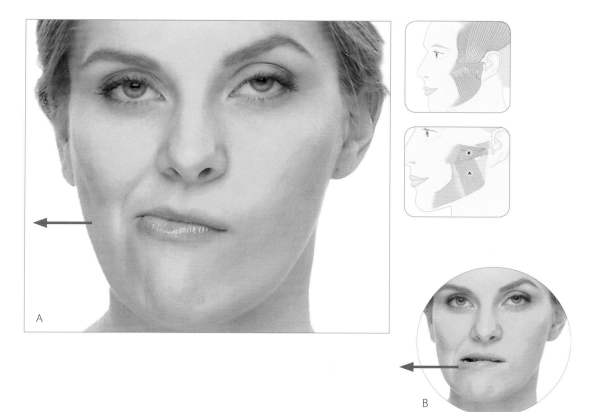

A

B

8 Coordinated jaw side-to-side exercise with tongue

a) Shift your jaw to the side and move your tongue to the same side, the tongue tip reaching the tooth farthest back in your upper jaw. Hold the position for 3–5 seconds. Return slowly. Do the same on the other side. Alternate this 5 times on both sides.

b) Average normal sideways movement of the jaw varies between 8 mm and 12 mm.

IMPACT ON HEALTH: Strengthens and relaxes the chewing muscles that move the lower jaw side to side.

STRETCHING TECHNIQUES
FOR THE CHEWING MUSCLES

The stretching techniques of MimiLift Facial MuscleCare aim to regain and maintain the optimal length of the chewing muscles. Appropriate stretches improve the healthy range of motion of the lower jaw and relieve tension and pain caused by tigthened chewing muscles.

Benefits

Tensed, tightened chewing muscles result in a stiff jaw and may cause local tenderness and referred pain to other locations. Remedial stretches relax and loosen the jaw and alleviate soreness and pain.

Tight, shortened chewing muscles restrict the mouth and jaw opening. Appropriate lengthening of the jaw-closing chewing muscles will increase the range of motion of the jaw into the physiologically ideal range.

Tight chewing muscles overload and put pressure on the jaw joints and cause faulty movements. Stretching releases the harmful pressure and restores the normal function of the jaw joints.

Tightened chewing muscles may lead over time to incorrect bite (occlusion) by changing the rest position of the lower jaw. Appropriate lengthening of the chewing muscles allows the lower jaw to find its best rest position and corrects the bite.

INSTRUCTIONS

- Perform all the stretches slowly and gently.
- Concentrate on the stretch.
- Stretch the chewing muscles carefully to a point of mild discomfort and hold the stretch for a while. The discomfort should begin to fade during the stretch, when the stretch gradually relieves tension and loosens your chewing muscles.
- Keep the muscles you are stretching relaxed. Breathing deliberately during the stretching helps you relax and control the stretches. Enjoy the relaxing feeling of stretches.
- If a stretch feels too uncomfortable and tenses your muscles, decrease the force or the range of movement or both.
- The feeling of the stretch should not be painful. It should not produce pain in the muscles or in the joints. Distinguish the feeling of a healthy muscle stretch from the sensation of pain.
- Hold each stretch for the recommended time and repeat each stretch the recommended number of times. You can increase the duration of a stretch as well the number of repetitions if you like and as long as it feels comfortable.
- Application of moist heat or cold is sometimes a helpful relaxing procedure before the stretching of the chewing muscles.

  CAUTION: Never perform sudden and forceful movements during stretching or try to force your jaw beyond its physiological limits. Those with a history of a jaw dislocation must be careful not to perform jaw movements that are too wide.

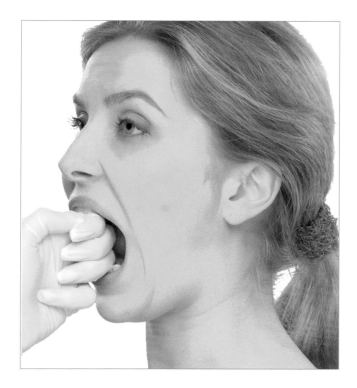

Jaw opening test

The maximum opening of the mouth and lower jaw in most individuals is more than 40 mm. The range of opening is slightly limited if the opening capacity is between 30–39 mm and severely restricted if it remains less than 30 mm (Helkimo index).

You can test your jaw opening by yourself. Your jaw opening is good if you can comfortably insert the first three knuckles of your non-dominant hand between your front teeth. If your opened jaws admit only two knuckles, your jaw opening is slightly limited. If you can get only one or one-half knuckles between your front teeth, your mouth opening is severely limited.

Stretching the jaw-closing muscles will regain the normal the jaw opening when a muscular problem is the underlying cause of the limited jaw opening.

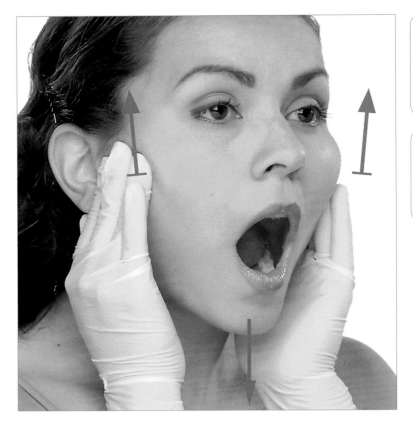
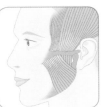
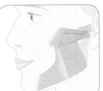

1 Dynamic stretch for the chewing muscles

Press your fingers firmly below your zygomatic arch. Lower your jaw slowly as far as you can while pressing your fingers very firmly against the skin and pushing upwards the soft tissues of the masseter muscle and zygomatic arch area. Hold this position for 5 seconds. Return gradually to the starting postion. Repeat 5 times.

IMPACT ON HEALTH: Relaxes and lengthens jaw-closing chewing muscles, especially masseter muscle. Strengthens jaw-opening muscles.
IMPACT ON APPEARANCE: Lifts the cheek area.

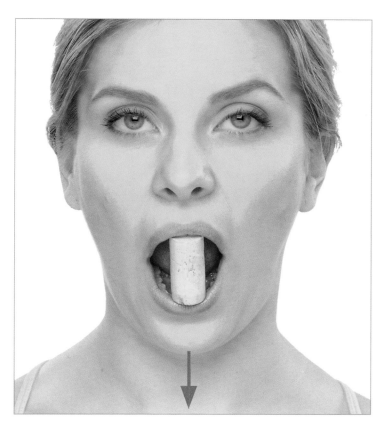

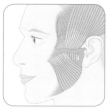

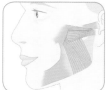

2 Intensive stretch for the chewing muscles

Place gently and carefully a cork or something similar of a suitable size and safe material between your teeth. Relax. Hold the stretch for 20–30 seconds and repeat the stretch 4 times. You may stretch even longer, but the maximum time to hold each stretch is one minute.

IMPACT ON HEALTH: This is an important stretch to lengthen all the jaw-closing chewing muscles and to increase the jaw opening. Helps speech and swallowing.

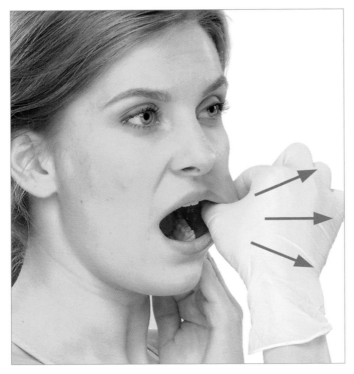
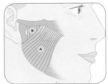

3 Stretching the chewing muscles from inside the mouth

Put your thumb inside your mouth. Push the cheek outwards with the thumb. Push the cheek with the thumb alternately diagonally downwards, straight to the side and diagonally upwards.

Open your jaw slowly during every stretch, and leave the jaw in the position where you feel the stretch best. Hold the stretch positions for 10 seconds and return to the starting position between the stretches. Repeat the stretches on the other side of your face. Repeat twice on both sides.

Use hygienic protective gloves or you may perform the stretches while taking a shower.

IMPACT ON HEALTH: This manually assisted stretch effectively relaxes and lengthens the jaw-closing chewing muscles in the cheek area, mainly the masseter muscle.
IMPACT ON APPEARANCE: Relaxed chewing muscles in the cheek area will give the cheeks the appearance of youthful roundness.

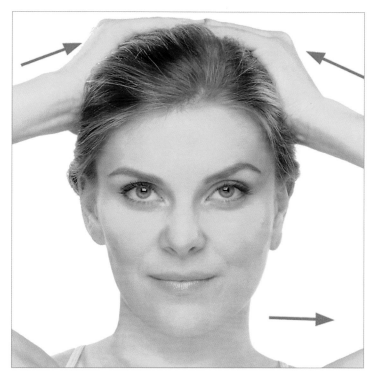

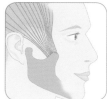

4 Stretching technique for the temporalis muscle

Press your palms very firmly against the sides of your head and interlock the fingers of both hands on the top of your head. Keep pressing and stretch the temporalis muscle by pulling it with your palms upward, alternately straight upwards and diagonally front and back. Hold each stretch position for 5 seconds. Repeat each stretch 2 times. Change the place of your palms slightly in the temporal area between the stretches.

In order to increase the feeling of the stretch in your temporal area, you may move your jaw to the side during the stretch or tilt your head sideways or down toward your chest.

IMPACT ON HEALTH: Releases tension in the temporalis muscle. Promotes a relaxed and optimal rest position of the jaw.

MASSAGE FOR THE CHEWING MUSCLES

Massage reduces tension, pain and tightness in the chewing muscles. It relaxes the chewing muscles in a pleasant way and promotes a sense of a general wellbeing.

Benefits

Massage mobilizes the stiff tissues of the chewing muscles. Massage techniques apply multidirectional stretching to the fascias and cells of the tight chewing muscles, relieving muscle stiffness.

Sustained contraction of the chewing muscles inititates local muscle pain and even referred pain to a larger area. When muscle tenderness and soreness is the main problem, pain relief can be achieved by gentle manual massage.

Massage increases local blood flow in the chewing muscles. The increased blood circulation brings more oxygen to the tissues and flushes the tissues of waste products and local chemical mediators of pain, all of which helps to relieve pain. Massage also eliminates local sore points of the chewing muscles.

Massage releases feel-good hormones and stimulates the nervous system to suppress the pain. Pain of the chewing muscles reduces and the chewing muscles relax. A sense of a general wellbeing ensues.

INSTRUCTIONS

- Massage of the chewing muscles should be painless but must be firm enough to remould the muscles and fascias.
- Choose a comfortable massage position in order to keep your hands and shoulders relaxed.
- You can vary the position of your hands as long as the massage technique remains the same. The most comfortable position is one where the wrists and fingers need to bend as little as possible.
- Perform the massage on clean skin without oil or any other lubricant.
- Wash your hands thoroughly before you begin to massage your facial area.
- Be careful not to scratch yourself with your fingernails.
- Repeat each massage stroke according to the recommended number of times or longer if necessary, until the treated muscles feel more relaxed.

CAUTION: Refrain from massage if there is an infection, an acute injury or a malign tumour in the facial area.

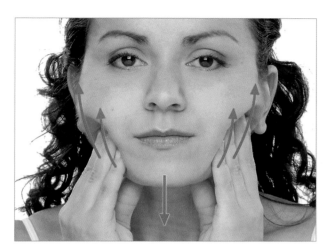

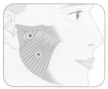

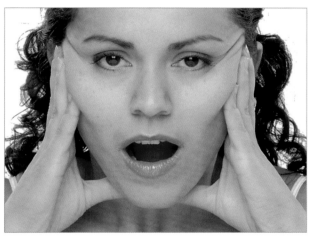

1 Longitudinal massage stroke for the masseter muscle

Press your fingers to the jaw angle. Push fingers very firmly and slowly upwards along the masseter muscle. This gliding massage stroke proceeds to the zygomatic arch. Open your jaw while the massage stroke proceeds. Repeat the massage stroke 6 times.

IMPACT ON HEALTH: Relaxes jaw-closing chewing muscles. Relieves tension and pain in the masseter muscle. Activates jaw-opening muscles.

IMPACT ON APPEARANCE: Lifts the cheek area.

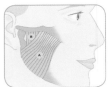

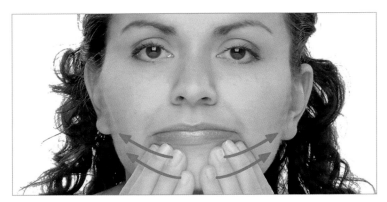

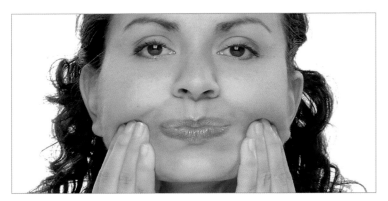

2 Transverse massage stroke for the masseter muscle

In the starting position, place your fingers against your chin. Glide your fingers slowly, evenly and very firmly from the chin straight to the side, all the way to the jaw angle.

The massage stroke glides across the masseter muscle and also over the mimic muscles of the lower face. Maintain firm pressure. Jut out the lips while the fingers proceed towards the jaw angle.

The first stroke goes close to the jaw line. Perform the next stroke slightly higher, starting closer to the corners of your mouth.

Repeat the massage strokes altogether 6 times.

IMPACT ON HEALTH: Relaxes the masseter muscle and also the mimic muscles of the lower face.

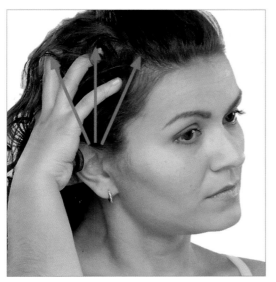

A

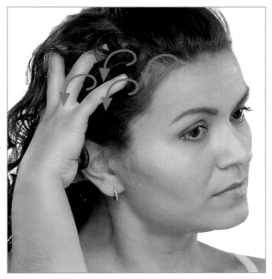

B

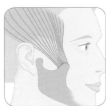

3 Gliding and friction strokes for the temporalis muscle

a) Spread your fingers slightly and place your fingertips on the side of your head, near your ear. Pressing firmly, glide your fingertips slowly along the temporalis muscle alternately straight upwards and diagonally upwards and backwards.

Keep your jaw a little open while the gliding stroke proceeds. Repeat the massage strokes altogether 6 times. Cover the entire temporalis muscle with the gliding strokes. Do the same massage to the other side of your head.

b) Apply firm circular pressures to the side of your head. Your fingertips do not slide over the muscle but move and loosen the temporalis muscle. Do four circles in each position. Repeat the friction stroke until you have covered the entire temporalis muscle. Keep your jaw a little open during the massage. Repeat the massage on the other side of your head.

IMPACT ON HEALTH: Relieves tension headache.

STRENGTHENING EXERCISES FOR THE **MIMIC MUSCLES**

MimiLift strengthening exercises target those muscles of the face that, when well-toned, contribute to lifting facial features and adding volume to the face. Strongly founded on anatomy and physiology, MimiLift provides an all-round conditioning and toning routine for the face, suitable for both beauty and health care.

Benefits

The strengthening exercises of MimiLift Facial MuscleCare challenge the muscles of the facial area to perform effective movements in the widest possible range of motion available to them. This activates large numbers of motor units in the facial muscles, which in turn builds the proportion of active muscle tissue. With the size of the individual muscle cells in the muscle growing, facial muscularity becomes stronger, firmer and plumper.

The MimiLift exercises also strengthen the fascial attachments and ligamentous support. Strong facial fascias and ligaments, together with firm, well-conditioned facial muscles, reduce facial sag and create a perfect, healthy and natural facelift.

MimiLift strengthening exercises put necessary stress on facial bones to strengthen the facial bone density. Good facial bone density slows down age-related general facial bone shrinkage as well as changes to the bone shape, which prevent soft tissue sagging due to better bone support.

The MimiLift strengthening exercise sequence is rigorously based on the anatomy and physiology of the mimic muscles, which make it well suited for restoring, improving and maintaining the normal motor functions of the mimic muscles.

INSTRUCTIONS

- Focus on the facial muscles that you are working on and keep the other muscles relaxed.
- Use the full range of motion.
- Perform all exercises carefully, slowly, smoothly and evenly to achieve the best results.
- The manual resistance resists gently but firmly the active movement without stopping it. It is helpful to wear thin gloves to prevent the grip from slipping.
- Keep your tongue close to your front teeth. Let your upper teeth separate slightly from the lower teeth to prevent undue strain when performing the exercises.
- Maintain a good upper body posture with the head well-aligned when doing the exercises.
- In the beginning you may use a mirror to guide you when learning the exercises, and you may use your finger to lightly guide the direction of the muscle movements.
- Repeat each exercise at least the recommended number of times. You can also increase the number of repetitions if you like.

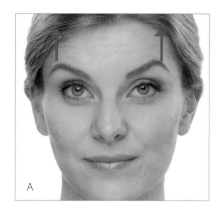

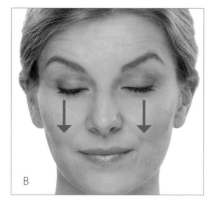

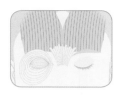

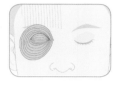

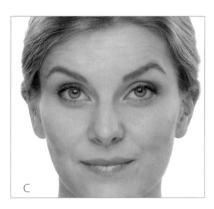

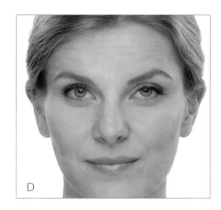

FOREHEAD AND EYE AREA

1 Combination exercise to strengthen the frontalis and orbicularis oculi muscles

a) Lift your eyebrows. b) Close your eyes. c) Open your eyes. d) Lower your eyebrows.

Concentrate on lifting the outer parts of your eyebrows in particular. Close your eyes firmly, without screwing them up. Repeat the whole sequence 10 times.

IMPACT ON APPEARANCE: Lifts the eyebrows and upper eyelids.
IMPACT ON HEALTH: Enhances facial muscle activity in functional patterns.

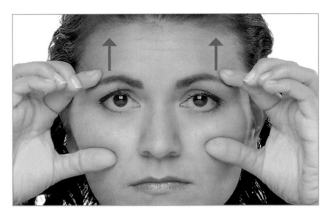

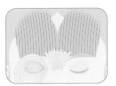

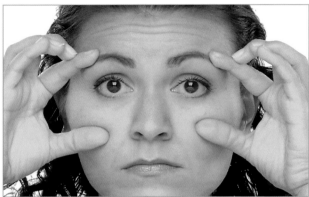

FOREHEAD

2 Resistance exercise to strengthen the frontalis muscle

Place your index fingers or the tips of three fingers above the outside part of your eyebrows. Press them firmly against the skin. Lift your eyebrows as high as you can and use your fingers to resist the lifting of the eyebrows.

Work smoothly, focusing on lifting the outer edges of the eyebrows. The resistance subtly resists the active movement through the full range of motion, without stopping the movement. Repeat 20 times.

IMPACT ON APPEARANCE: Intensified lifting of the lateral eyebrows.

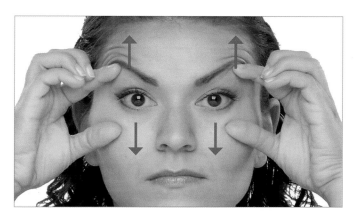

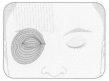

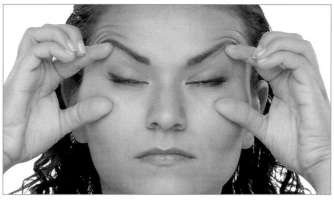

EYE AREA

3 Resistance exercise to strengthen the orbicularis oculi muscle

Lift your eyebrows and place your index fingers under the outer edges of the eyebrows and the thumbs under the outer corner of the eyes. Press them firmly against the skin and use your index fingers to keep the eyebrows lifted.

Close and open your eyes. Close your eyes slowly each time, and keep them firmly closed for a short moment. Repeat 20 times.

IMPACT ON APPEARANCE: Intensified lifting and toning of the upper eyelids.

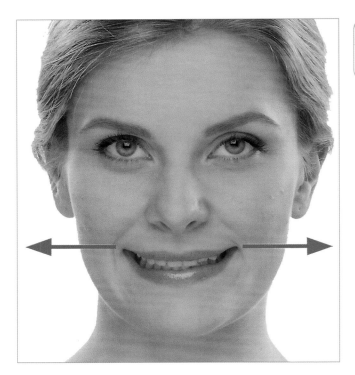

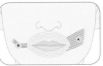

LOWER CHEEK

1 Basic exercise to strengthen the buccinator and risorius muscles

Pull the corners of mouth straight sideways. Maintain for a while in the extreme position before returning to the starting position. Keep the movements slow, even and smooth. Concentrate on the exercise. Use the muscles of your cheek. Keep the rest of your facial muscles relaxed. Repeat 20 times.

Let your tongue rest close to your front teeth and let your upper teeth separate from the lower teeth slightly to prevent undue strain when performing the exercise.

IMPACT ON APPEARANCE: Tones the lower cheek.
IMPACT ON HEALTH: Enhances facial muscle activity in functional patterns.

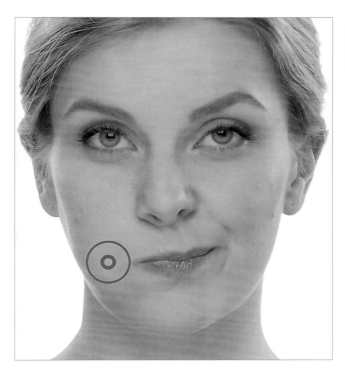

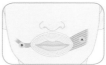

LOWER CHEEK

2 Basic exercise to strengthen the buccinator muscle

Puff out your right cheek. Puff out your left cheek. Hold the air in for a little while in each side. Repeat 5 times on both sides.

IMPACT ON APPEARANCE: Tones the lower cheek.
IMPACT ON HEALTH: Enhances facial muscle activity in functional patterns.

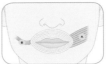

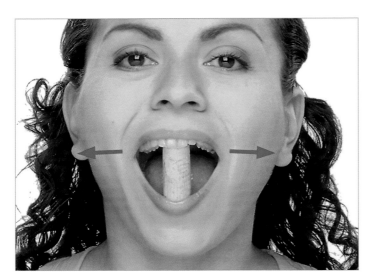

LOWER CHEEK

3 Combination exercise to strengthen the buccinator and risorius muscles

Place a cork or something similar of a suitable size between your teeth to keep your lower jaw down. Hold the position and simultaneously pull the corners of mouth straight sideways.

Repeat 10 times. Close your mouth and rest for a few seconds. Place the cork again and repeat another 10 times.

IMPACT ON APPEARANCE: Tones the lower cheek.
IMPACT ON HEALTH: Relaxes and lengthens jaw-closing chewing muscles.

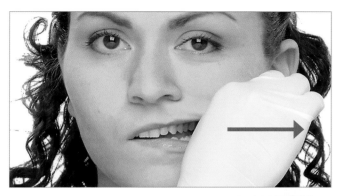

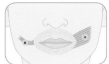

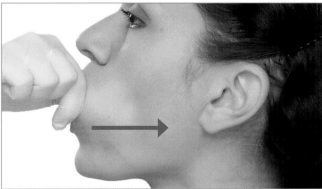

LOWER CHEEK

4 Resistance exercise to strengthen the buccinator and risorius muscles

Grip near the corner of the mouth using a solid pinching action. Pull the corner of the mouth slowly straight to the side while your fingers gently resist the movement through the whole range of motion.

The resistance subtly resists the active movement through the full range of motion, without stopping the movement. Keep in the extreme position for a while and return slowly to the starting position. Repeat 20 times on both sides.

IMPACT ON APPEARANCE: Intensified toning of the lower cheek.

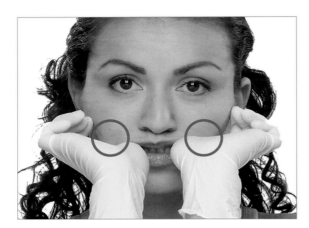

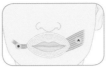

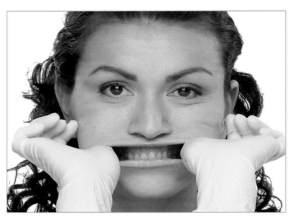

LOWER CHEEK

5 Resistance exercise to strengthen the buccinator muscle

Place your thumbs inside your mouth, against the wall of your cheeks, horizontally at the level of the corners of your mouth. At first push the cheeks outwards with your thumbs, and then begin to slowly compress the cheeks inward while your thumbs firmly resist the movement through the whole range of motion. Repeat 20 times.

IMPACT ON APPEARANCE: Intensified toning of the lower cheek.

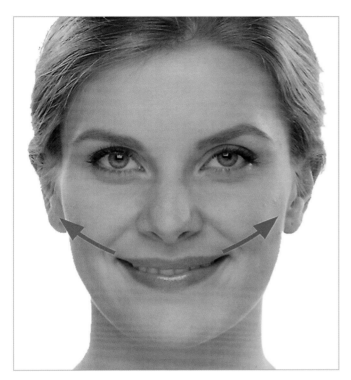

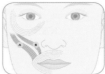

UPPER CHEEK

1 Basic exercise to strengthen the zygomaticus major and zygomaticus minor muscles

Pull the corners of your mouth towards your ears. Maintain for a while in the extreme position before returning to the starting position. Concentrate on elavating the musculature covering your cheekbones. Repeat 20 times.

IMPACT ON APPEARANCE: Lifts the upper cheek.
IMPACT ON HEALTH: Enhances facial muscle activity in functional patterns.

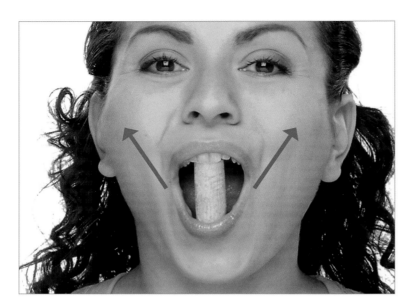

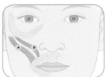

UPPER CHEEK

2 Combination exercise to strengthen the zygomaticus major and zygomaticus minor muscles

Place a cork or something similar of a suitable size between your teeth to keep your lower jaw down. Hold the position and simultaneously pull the corners of your mouth towards your ears. Repeat 10 times.

Close your mouth and rest for a few seconds. Place the cork again and repeat another 10 times.

IMPACT ON APPEARANCE: Lifts the upper cheek.
IMPACT ON HEALTH: Relaxes and lengthens jaw-closing chewing muscles.

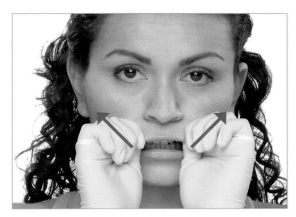

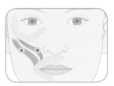

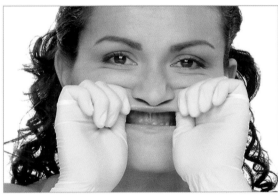

UPPER CHEEK

3 Resistance exercise to strengthen the zygomaticus major and zygomaticus minor muscles

Grip just above the corners of your mouth using a solid pinching action. Pull the corners of your mouth towards your ears while your fingers gently resist the movement through the whole range of motion. Keep in the extreme position for a while and return slowly to the starting position.

The resistance subtly resists the active movement through the full range of motion, without stopping the movement. Repeat 20 times.

IMPACT ON APPEARANCE: Intensified lifting of the upper cheek.

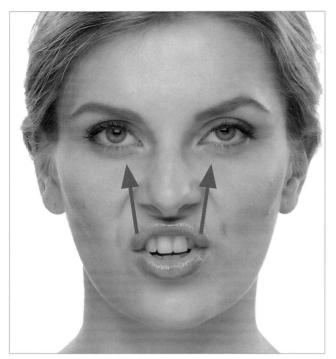

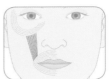

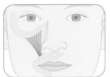

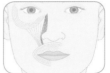

MIDFACE

1 Basic exercise to strengthen the levator anguli oris, levator labii superioris and levator labii superioris alaeque nasi muscles

Raise your upper lip upward. Maintain for a while in the extreme position before returning to the starting position. Concentrate on elavating the musculature of your midface. Repeat 20 times.

IMPACT ON APPEARANCE: Lifts the midface. (The midface is the area between the lower eyelid and the mouth.)
IMPACT ON HEALTH: Enhances facial muscle activity in functional patterns.

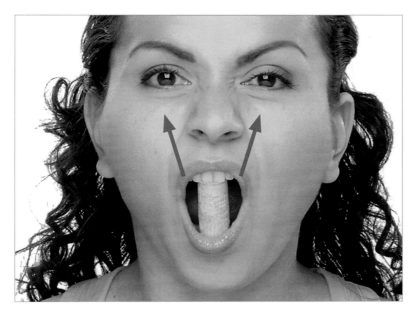
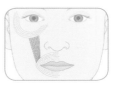
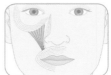
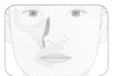

MIDFACE

2 Combination exercise to strengthen the levator anguli oris, levator labii superioris and levator labii superioris alaeque nasi muscles

Place a cork or something similar of a suitable size between your teeth to keep your lower jaw down. Hold the position and simultaneously raise your upper lip upwards.

Repeat 10 times. Close your mouth and rest for a few seconds. Place the cork again and repeat another 10 times. Concentrate on elavating the musculature of your midface.

IMPACT ON APPEARANCE: Lifts the midface.
IMPACT ON HEALTH: Relaxes and lengthens jaw-closing chewing muscles.

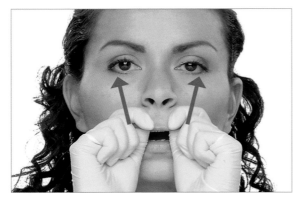

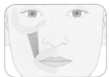

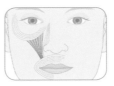

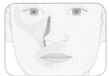

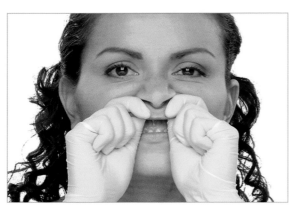

MIDFACE

3 Resistance exercise to strengthen the levator anguli oris, levator labii superioris and levator labii superioris alaeque nasi muscles

Grip above your upper lip using a solid pinching action. Raise your upper lip towards your nose while your fingers gently resist the movement through the whole range of motion.

Remain in the extreme position for a while and return slowly to the starting position. Concentrate on elavating the musculature of your midface. Repeat 20 times.

IMPACT ON APPEARANCE: Intensified lifting of the midface.

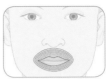

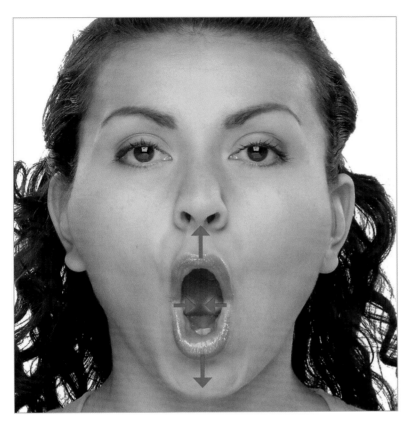

LIPS

1 Basic exercise to strengthen the orbicularis oris muscle

Open your mouth, jut out your lips and draw the corners of your mouth towards each other. Hold the position for a while. Close your mouth. Repeat 10 times.

IMPACT ON APPEARANCE: Restores fullness to the lips.
IMPACT ON HEALTH: Enhances facial muscle activity in functional patterns.

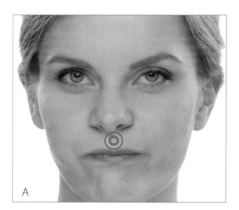

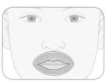

A

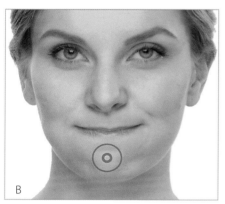

B

LIPS

2 Basic exercise to strengthen the orbicularis oris muscle

a) Puff out your upper lip. Hold the air in for a little while under your upper lip.
b) Puff out your lower lip. Hold the air in for a little while under your lower lip.
Repeat 5 times in both positions.

IMPACT ON APPEARANCE: Restores fullness to the lips.
IMPACT ON HEALTH: Enhances facial muscle activity in functional patterns.

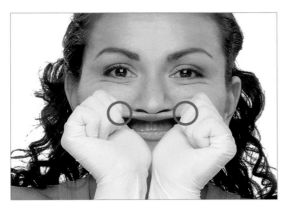

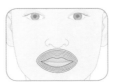

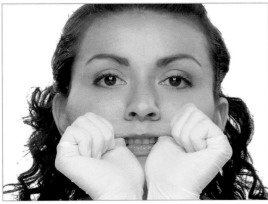

LIPS

3 Resistance exercise to strengthen the upper region of the orbicularis oris muscle

Place your thumbs diagonally under your upper lip. First push your upper lip outwards and diagonally upwards and then begin to slowly pull the upper lip down while your thumbs firmly resist the movement through the whole range of motion. Repeat 20 times.

IMPACT ON APPEARANCE: Intensified plumping of the upper lip.

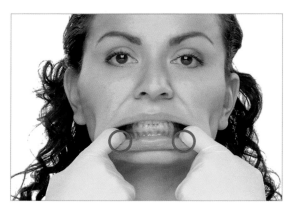

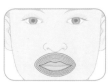

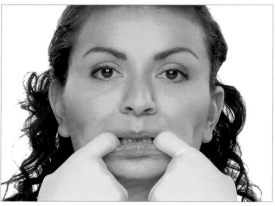

LIPS

4 Resistance exercise to strengthen the lower region of the orbicularis oris muscle

Place your index fingers diagonally under your lower lip. First push your lower lip gently outwards and then begin to slowly pull the upper lip up while your index fingers firmly resist the movement through the whole range of motion. Repeat 20 times.

IMPACT ON APPEARANCE: Intensified plumping of the lower lip.

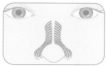

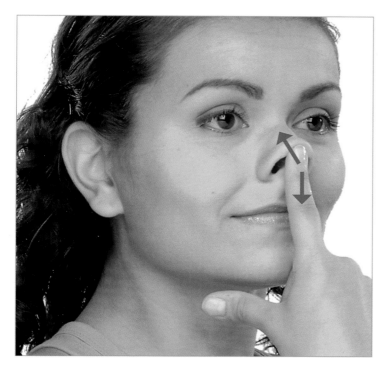

NOSE

1 Resistance exercise to strengthen the muscles of the nose

Push the tip of your nose upward with your finger. Keep your nose tip up like this while you try to pull it down with the muscles of your nose. The actual movement is very small because your finger is preventing it. You rhythmically tense the muscles of your nose during the repetions. Repeat 10 times.

IMPACT ON APPEARANCE: Lifts the nose tip.

RELAXING TECHNIQUES FOR THE MIMIC MUSCLES

Tension and tightness in the mimic muscles result in lines in the skin of the face and may cause discomfort and pain. By following the precise stretching and massage techniques of MimiLift Facial MucleCare you will be able to remove excess tension, which smooths out facial lines and creases and alleviates muscle-related facial pains and headaches.

Benefits

Unpleasant and harmful muscle tension and tightness in the facial area can be relieved by the unique MimiLift massage and stretching techniques. These relaxing procedures penetrate the surface of the skin, thus remoulding the underlying muscles. They apply multidirectional stretching to the taut muscles and thus relieve muscle stiffness. Relaxation of the mimic muscles smooths out lines and creases and reduces their formation. MimiLift Facial MuscleCare is a revolutionary, totally non-invasive line-smoothing method.

Facial relaxation is vital for facial health as it eliminates muscle-based facial pains and headaches. It is needed for good voice production and it may be helpful in stuttering. Proper stretching and massage techniques also relieve and prevent stiffness, tightness and spasms of the mimic muscles due to neurological problems.

Mimic muscles are connected to emotions. A relaxed face promotes your own wellbeing by causing overall relaxation. A relaxed face gives also a positive impression to the person you are communicating with.

INSTRUCTIONS

- The massage should not be painful, but the strokes should be firm enough to remould the muscles and fascias underneath the skin of the face.
- Perform the massage on clean skin without oil or any other lubricant.
- Perform all the stretches slowly and gently and concentrate on the stretch.
- In techniques where the grip should not slip it is helpful to wear thin gloves or use a piece of soft fabric.
- Choose comfortable positions in order to keep your hands and shoulders relaxed. You can vary the position of your hands as long as the massage or manual stretching technique remains the same. The most comfortable position is one where the wrists and fingers need to bend as little as possible.
- Wash your hands thoroughly before you begin to touch your facial area.
- Be careful not to scratch yourself with your fingernails.
- Repeat each massage stroke and hold each stretch as recommended or you may increase the repetitions and durations until the treated muscles feel more relaxed.
  CAUTION: Please refrain from massage and manual stretching if there is an infection, an acute injury or a malign tumour in the facial area.

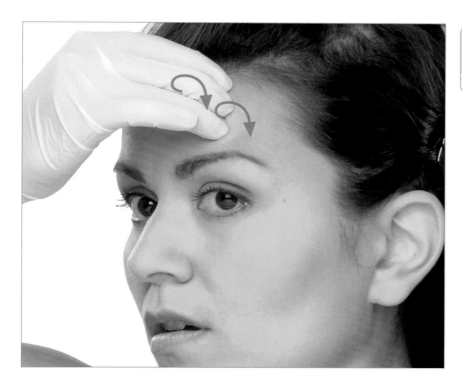
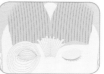

FOREHEAD

1 Friction stroke for the frontalis muscle

Apply firm circular pressures to your forehead. The fingertips do not slide over the skin but move and loosen the forehead's muscle under the skin. The friction stroke proceeds from the middle of the forehead to the sides. Do 4 circles in each place. Repeat the procedure until you have covered every part of your forehead.

PROCEDURE: Relaxing the forehead's frontalis muscle.

IMPACT ON HEALTH: Relieves tension headache.

IMPACT ON APPEARANCE: Diminishes horizontal forehead creases.

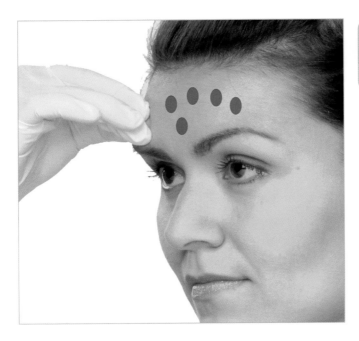

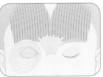

FOREHEAD

2 Pinching stroke for the frontalis muscle

Carefully squeeze the frontalis muscle underneath the skin of the forehead using a pinching action. Keep lifting the small amount of muscle and pinch it lightly few times between your fingers or move it gently back and forth or with circular motion using very small movements. Repeat few times in each place.

Proceed from the side of your forehead to the middle, and also treat the area between the eyebrows. Work especially on areas where forehead's creases exist. In places where your forehead is very tight, do not try to use the pinching stroke by force. Wear thin gloves or use a piece of soft fabric to prevent the grip from slipping.

PROCEDURE: Relaxing the forehead's frontalis muscle.

IMPACT ON HEALTH: Relieves tension headache.

IMPACT ON APPEARANCE: Diminishes horizontal forehead creases.

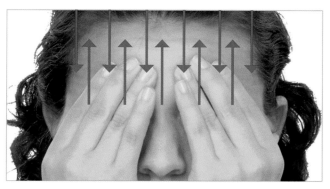

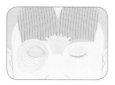

A, B

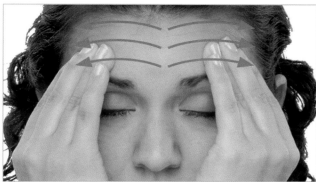

C

FOREHEAD

3 Gliding strokes for the frontalis muscle

Slide your fingers slowly and firmly with pressure, first a) widely from the hairline to the middle of your forehead, then b) from above your eyebrows upwards to the hairline, and finally c) from the middle of your forehead to the sides.

Repeat each stroke few times, and cover your entire forehead with the firm, calm, gliding strokes.

PROCEDURE: Relaxes the forehead's frontalis muscle.

IMPACT ON HEALTH: Relieves tension headache.

IMPACT ON APPEARANCE: Diminishes horizontal forehead creases.

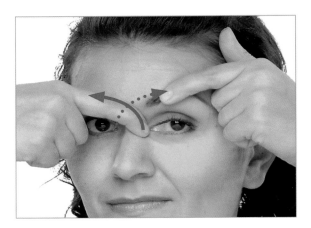

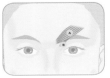

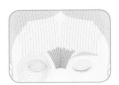

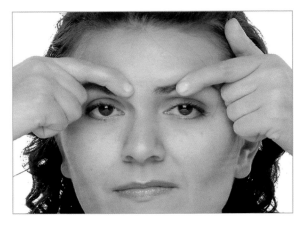

PROCEDURE: Relaxes the corrugator supercilii muscle, depressor supercilii muscle and the procerus muscle.

IMPACT ON HEALTH: The branch of the trigeminal nerve that penetrates the corrugator supercilii muscle may get pinched if this muscle is tight and tensed. Relaxation of the corrugator supercilii muscle helps in migraine-type headache caused by this nerve entrapment.

IMPACT ON APPEARANCE: Relaxation of the corrugator supercilii and depressor supercilii muscles smooths out vertical furrows, or 'frown lines', between the eyebrows. Relaxation of the procerus muscle smooths out transverse creases at the nasal bridge.

AREA BETWEEN THE EYEBROWS

1 Gliding stroke for all the muscles between the eyebrows

Pull firmly with your index finger from the inner corner of the eye, across the area between the eyebrows, just above the middle of the eyebrow. Do the same massage on the other side with your other hand. Continue alternating these gliding strokes a few times on both sides.

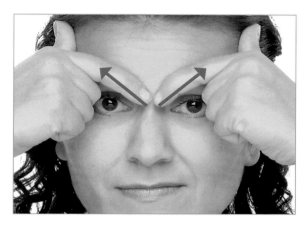

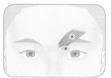

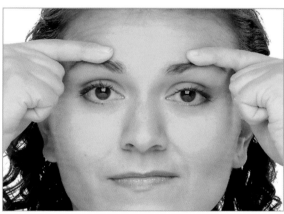

PROCEDURE: Relaxes the corrugator supercilii muscle and depressor supercilii muscle.

IMPACT ON HEALTH: The branch of the trigeminal nerve that penetrates the corrugator supercilii muscle may get pinched if this muscle is tight and tensed. Relaxation of the corrugator supercilii muscle helps in migraine-type headache caused by this nerve entrapment.

IMPACT ON APPEARANCE: Relaxation of the corrugator supercilii muscle and depressor supercilii muscles smooths out vertical furrows between the eyebrows.

AREA BETWEEN THE EYEBROWS

2 Gliding stroke for the corrugator supercilii muscle

Press the index fingers to the root of the nose. The index fingers glide firmly with moderate pressure along the corrugator supercilii muscle, from the root of the nose diagonally upwards, just above to the middle of both eyebrows. Repeat several times, working evenly and slowly.

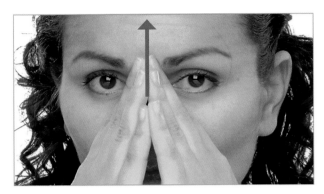

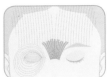

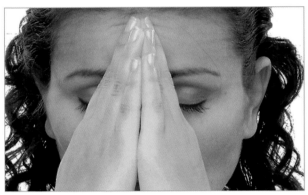

AREA BETWEEN THE EYEBROWS

3 Gliding stroke for the procerus muscle

Place your index fingers to the bridge of your nose. Glide your index fingers firmly with moderate pressure along the procerus muscle, from the bridge of the nose up towards the hairline. Repeat several times, working evenly and slowly.

PROCEDURE: Relaxes the procerus muscle.

IMPACT ON HEALTH: Relieves tension headache.

IMPACT ON APPEARANCE: Relaxation of the procerus muscle smooths out transverse creases at the nasal bridge.

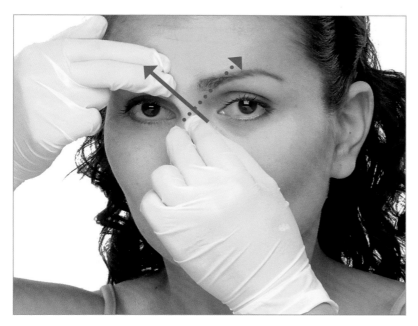

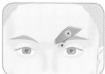

AREA BETWEEN THE EYEBROWS

4a Stretching technique for the corrugator supercilii muscle

Take hold of the attachment of the corrugator supercilii muscle in the root of the nose. Place the fingers of your other hand above the medial part of the eyebrow and stretch the corrugator muscle by pulling it diagonally upwards. Hold the stretch for a while and do the same to the other side. Wear thin gloves or use a piece of soft fabric to prevent the grip from slipping.

PROCEDURE: Relaxes the corrugator supercilii muscle and depressor supercilii muscle.

IMPACT ON APPEARANCE: Relaxation of the corrugator supercilii muscle and depressor supercilii muscle smooths out vertical furrows between the eyebrows.

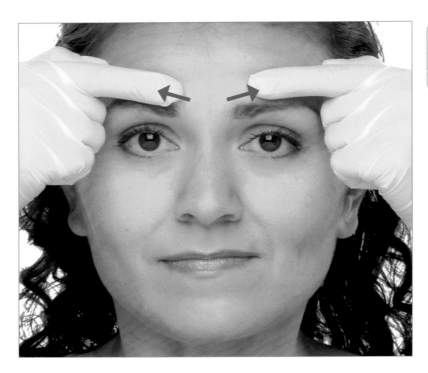

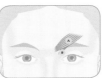

AREA BETWEEN THE EYEBROWS

4b Stretching technique for the corrugator supercilii muscle

Press your fingers just above the medial part of the eyebrows. Stretch the corrugator supercilii muscles by pulling with the fingers to the opposite directions. Hold the stretch for a few seconds and repeat 2–4 times. Wear thin gloves or use a piece of soft fabric to prevent the grip from slipping.

PROCEDURE: Relaxes the corrugator supercilii muscle and depressor supercilii muscle.
IMPACT ON APPEARANCE: Relaxation of the corrugator supercilii muscle and depressor supercilii muscle smooths out vertical furrows between the eyebrows.

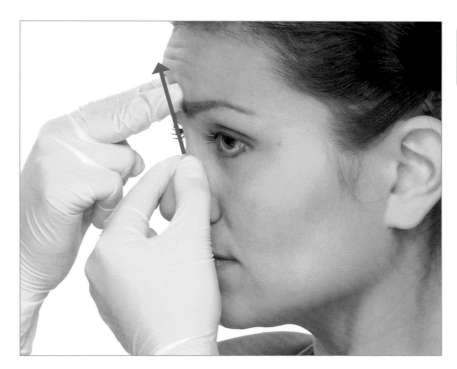

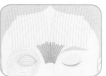

AREA BETWEEN THE EYEBROWS

5 Stretching technique for the procerus muscle

Stretch the procerus muscle by pushing it upwards towards the hairline with your fingers. The other hand keeps the hold of the attachment of the procerus muscle in the bridge of the nose. Hold the stretch for a few seconds and repeat 2–4 times. Wear thin gloves or use a piece of soft fabric to prevent the grip from slipping.

PROCEDURE: Relaxes the procerus muscle.
IMPACT ON APPEARANCE: Relaxation of the procerus muscle smooths out transverse creases at the nasal bridge.

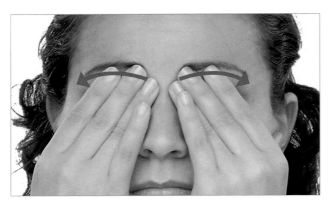

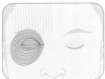

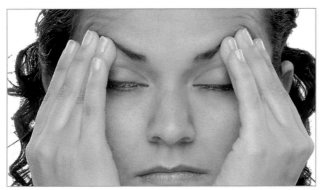

EYE AREA

1 Gliding stroke for the orbicularis oculi muscle

Place your fingertips under the inner edges of your eyebrows. Pressing firmly upward against the bony rim of the eye socket, slide your fingers right below the eyebrows to the lateral edge of the eyebrows.

As you perform the gliding stroke, your fingers elevate your eyebrows at the same time. Keep your eyes closed and avoid pressing your eyeballs. Repeat the gliding stroke several times.

> **PROCEDURE:** Relaxes the orbicularis oculi muscle.
> **IMPACT ON HEALTH:** Relaxes the eyes.
> **IMPACT ON APPEARANCE:** Elevates the eyebrows.

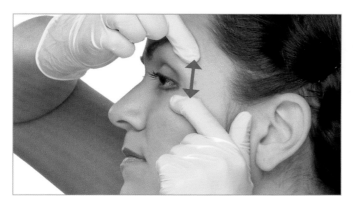

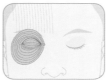

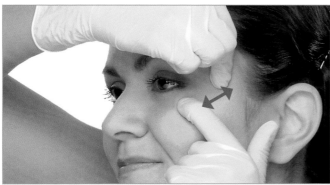

EYE AREA

2 Stretching technique for the orbicularis oculi muscle

Press your index fingers under the lateral edge of the eyebrow, a little apart from each other. Keep pressing the fingers firmly against the skin to prevent them from sliding. Stretch the orbicularis oculi muscle by pulling with fingers very gently in opposite directions.

Move downwards and repeat a similar stretch. Hold the stretch for a few seconds and repeat 2–4 times. Wear thin gloves or use a piece of soft fabric to prevent your fingers from slipping.

> **PROCEDURE:** Relaxes the orbicularis oculi muscle.
> **IMPACT ON HEALTH:** Relaxes the eyes.
> **IMPACT ON APPEARANCE:** Reduces fine lines around the eyes and elevates the lateral part of the eyebrows.

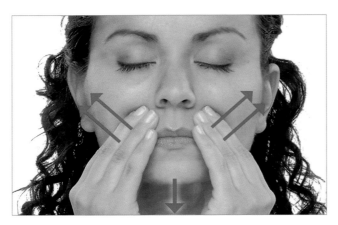
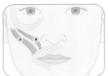

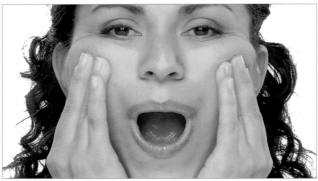

CHEEKBONE AREA

1 Gliding stroke for the cheekbone area

Slide your fingers firmly from near the corners of your mouth diagonally upwards and over your cheekbones. Open your jaw while the gliding stroke proceeds and lifts the soft tissues of the cheekbone area. Repeat a few times.

PROCEDURE: Relaxes the zygomaticus major and zygomaticus minor muscles.
IMPACT ON HEALTH: Promotes healthy voice production by removing tension from the muscles that move the lips.
IMPACT ON APPEARANCE: Lifts and volumizes the cheekbone area. Smooths out nose-to-mouth creases.

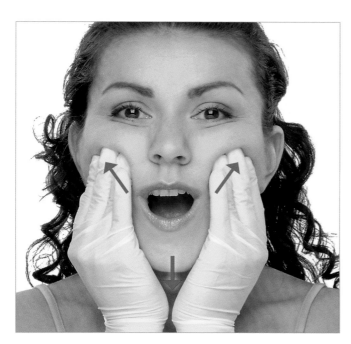
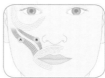

CHEEKBONE AREA

1 Stretching technique for the cheekbone area

Press your fingers below your cheekbones. Keep pressing the fingers very firmly against the skin and push the soft tissues of the cheekbone area upwards. At the same time open your jaw and draw the upper lip over the upper teeth. Hold the stretch for a few seconds and repeat 2–4 times.

PROCEDURE: Relaxes the zygomaticus major and zygomaticus minor muscles.
IMPACT ON HEALTH: Promotes healthy voice production by removing tension from the muscles that move the lips.
IMPACT ON APPEARANCE: Lifts and volumizes the cheekbone area. Smooths out nose-to-mouth creases.

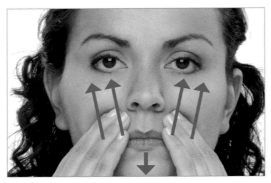

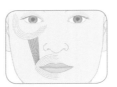

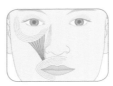

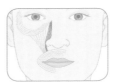

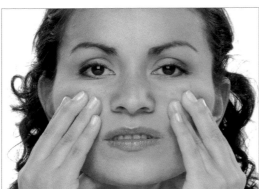

MIDFACE AREA

1 Gliding stroke for the midface area

Slide your fingers firmly against the skin from above your upper lip upwards to your cheekbones. Open your jaw while the gliding stroke proceeds and lifts the soft tissues of the midface area. Repeat several times.

PROCEDURE: Relaxes the levator anguli oris, levator labii superioris and levator labii superioris alaeque nasi muscles.

IMPACT ON HEALTH: Promotes healthy voice production by removing tension from the muscles that move the lips.

IMPACT ON APPEARANCE: Lifts and volumizes the midface area. Smooths out nose-to-mouth creases.

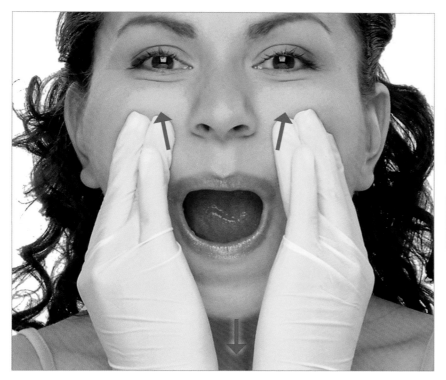

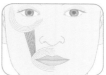

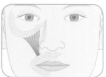

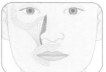

MIDFACE AREA

2 Stretching technique for the midface area

Press your fingers near the edges of your nostrils. Keep pressing the fingers very firmly against the skin and push the soft tissues of the midface area upwards. At the same time open your jaw and draw the upper lip over the upper teeth. Hold the stretch for a few seconds and repeat 2–4 times.

PROCEDURE: Relaxes the levator anguli oris, levator labii superioris and levator labii superioris alaeque nasi muscles.

IMPACT ON HEALTH: Promotes healthy voice production by removing tension from the muscles that move the lips.

IMPACT ON APPEARANCE: Lifts and volumizes the midface area. Smooths out nose-to-mouth creases.

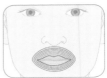

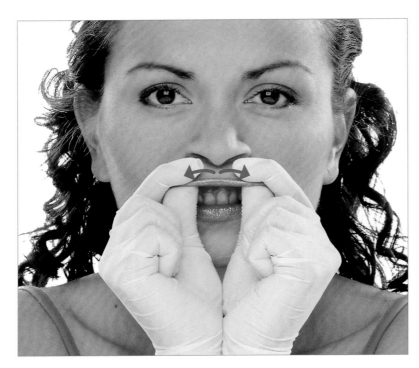

MOUTH AREA

1 Stretching technique for the orbicularis oris muscle

Take hold of the upper lip with a firm grip, thumbs inside the mouth and index fingers outside. Stretch the ring muscle of the mouth by pushing the upper lip at first slightly outwards and upwards and then by gently pulling the muscle with your fingers in the opposite direction.

Change the position of your fingers and do the same stretch along the whole upper lip. Stretch the lower lip in the same way. Hold each stretch for a few seconds and repeat twice.

Use thin, well-fitting, clean protective cloves. They are both hygienic and prevent the grip from slipping.

> **PROCEDURE:** Relaxes the orbicularis oris muscle.
> **IMPACT ON HEALTH:** Promotes healthy voice production by removing tension from the ring muscle of the mouth.
> **IMPACT ON APPEARANCE:** Smooths out vertical lip lines and restores the fullness of the lips.

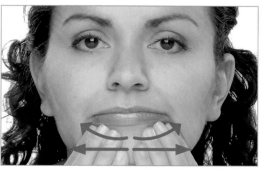
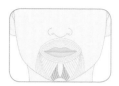
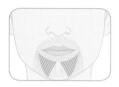
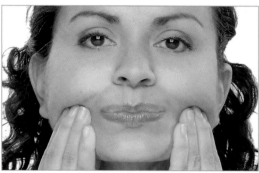
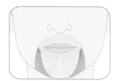

CHIN AREA

1 Gliding stroke for the chin area

a) Place your fingers in the middle of the chin under the lower lip. Keep pressing the fingers against the skin and slide the fingers first from the middle of the chin all the way to the jaw angle. Jut out your lips slightly while the fingers proceed. Repeat several times with firm and vigorous pressure.

b) Then slide the fingers from the middle of the chin diagonally upwards towards the corners of your mouth. Jut out your lips slightly while the fingers proceed. Repeat several times slowly and evenly.

PROCEDURE: Relaxes the mentalis, depressor labii inferioris and depressor anguli oris muscles.

IMPACT ON HEALTH: Promotes healthy voice production by removing tension from the muscles that move the lips.

IMPACT ON APPEARANCE: Diminishes chin crease and lines going down form the corners of the mouth.

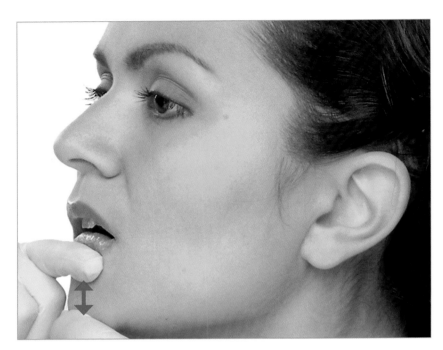

CHIN AREA

2 Stretching technique for the mentalis muscle

Press your index fingers firmly against your chin. Stretch the mentalis muscle by pulling it gently with the fingers in opposite directions. One fingers pushes upwards and the other pulls downwards.

Wear thin gloves or use a piece of soft fabric to prevent slipping. Hold the stretch for a few seconds and repeat 2–4 times.

PROCEDURE: Relaxes the mentalis muscle.
IMPACT ON APPEARANCE: Diminishes horizontal chin crease.

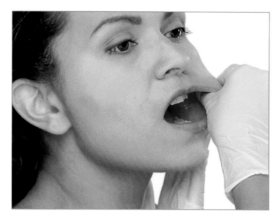

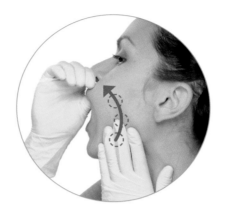

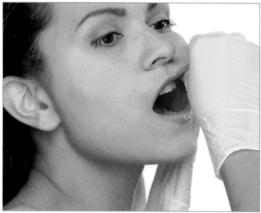

PROCEDURE: Relaxing the buccinator and risorius muscles and other mucles that attach to the corner of the mouth and upper lip.

IMPACT ON HEALTH: Promotes healthy voice production by removing tension from the muscles that move the lips.

IMPACT ON APPEARANCE: Restores fullness to the cheeks. Smooths out nose-to-mouth creases.

ENTIRE CHEEK

1 Stretching technique for the entire cheek

Put your thumb inside your mouth. Push your cheek gently outwards and upwards. Proceed in an arch motion from below the level of the corner of your mouth all the way up to the midface area. The other hand may support the jaw. Hold each stretch for a few seconds and repeat twice. Use hygienic protective gloves.

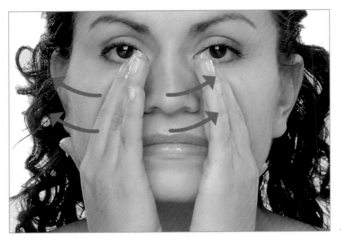

A

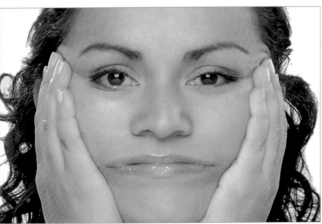

Finishing massage strokes

a) Slide your hands slowly and very gently from the middle of your face outwards and sideways in a long, light sweeping movement. Stop in front of your ears.

b) Change the direction of the light gliding stroke. Proceed downwards along the sides of your face.

c) Slide your fingers behind your ears.

d) The last light gliding stroke proceeds from behind the ears downwards along the neck, all the way to the collar bones.

Repeat 2–4 times. These light, long gliding strokes are used in the end of the session to sooth and relax.

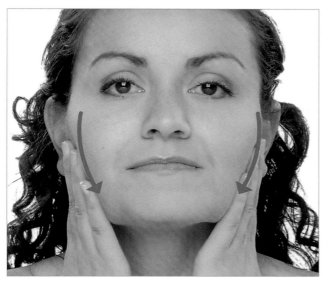

B

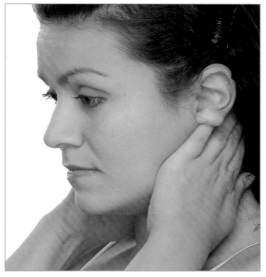

C

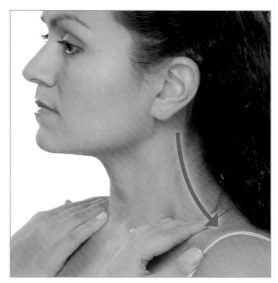

D

PHYSIOLOGICAL EFFECTS OF MIMILIFT

MimiLift Facial MuscleCare is a medically based method developed to look after the condition of the muscles of your face, jaw, head and neck. MimiLift Facial MuscleCare consists of precise stretching and massage techniques and relaxing and strenghtening exercises which impact not only on facial musculature but also on facial skin, fascias, ligaments, bones, jaw joints and the nervous system.

Relaxed facial musculature

Unfavourable muscle tightness and tension in the facial area can be relieved by the unique massage and stretching techniques of MimiLift Facial MuscleCare. These relaxing procedures penetrate the surface of the skin, thus remoulding the underlying muscles. They apply multidirectional stretching to the fibres of taut muscles and thus relieve muscle stiffness. As muscles and fascias cannot be separated, all stretching is myofascial stretching, and MimiLift Facial MuscleCare releases tension in the whole facial myofascial system. Relaxation of the mimic muscles smooths out lines and creases. Mimilift Facial MuscleCare is a revolutionary, totally non-invasive line-smoothing method.

Relaxed mimic and chewing muscles that retain their normal length and tone make facial features soft, giving the face a peaceful, pleasant look. Facial relaxation is vital for facial health as it eliminates muscle-based facial pains, headaches and teeth grinding and is necessary for good voice production. It may also be helpful in cases such as tinnitus, stuttering or sleep problems.

Well-conditioned facial musculature

The strengthening exercises of MimiLift Facial Muscle-Care challenge the muscles to perform the movements effectively in the widest possible range of motion available to them. This means that increasingly more motor units in the facial muscles are activated, which in turn increases the proportion of active muscle tissue. With the size of the individual muscle cells in the muscles increasing, facial muscularity becomes stronger and plumper. Well-toned facial muscles resist sagging, give a defined shape to the face and lift facial features. Good condition of mimic and chewing muscles will add youthful volume to the face and fill the space left from fat wasting.

The movement exercises of MimiLift Facial MuscleCare train the muscles of the facial area to function properly. Well-functioning jaw muscles are important in creating normal, healthy movements of the jaw and avoiding harmful muscle tension and unnatural strain on the jaw joints.

Strong facial bones, ligaments and fascias

Bones and ligaments need physical stress to remain strong. MimiLift Facial MuscleCare puts increased stress on facial bones, fascias and ligaments through strengthening exercises and precise facial soft tissue manipulation techniques. These procedures stimulate the bone-building cells (osteoblasts) to grow new bone. Good facial bone density slows down general age-related facial bone shrinkage as well as changes in the bone shape, which prevents soft tissue sagging due to better bone support.

The procedures of MimiLift Facial MuscleCare strengthen and remould also the facial fascias and ligaments. Strong yet elastic facial fascias and ligaments together with firm, well-conditioned facial musculature reduce facial sag and create a perfect natural facelift.

Healthy jaw joints

Cartilage tissues of the jaw joints need a certain amount of loading to remain healthy. Movements of the jaw joints function like a pump, bringing nutrients to the articular surfaces and removing waste products.

Gentle, controlled jaw movements produce a growth stimulus in the cartilage of the jaw joints, reduce pain and maintain the normal functions and range of motion of the jaw joints.

Glowing skin

MimiLift Facial MuscleCare stimulates blood circulation in the facial capillaries. Healthy pink glow of the skin is an obvious testament to improved blood flow. Improved circulation enhances the supply of oxygen and nutrients to facial muscles and renewing skin cells.

The procedures further stimulate lymphatic flow, which helps to flush away waste products and relieve puffiness of the face. The manual soft tissue techniques of MimiLift Facial MuscleCare stimulate fibroblast activity in the skin, promoting collagen and elastin production for a youthful skin and reduction of wrinkles.

Benefits for the nervous system

All MimiLift relaxing techniques serve to relax both mimic and chewing muscles by causing the brain to send relaxation-inducing signals to muscles to relieve tension and stiffness. MimiLift techniques make you more aware of any tension in your face, thus enabling you to avoid unnecessary straining of your face.

MimiLift exercises improve the recruitment of motor nerves in the face, which translates into an enhanced ability to control voluntary actions in the face. You will develop an improved awareness of your facial muscles, which enables you to avoid unfavourable facial habits and fixed facial expression patterns.

Mind and body have a reciprocal relationship, and especially facial muscles which are linked to emotions. Emotional conditions affect the face and the conditions of the face affect the mind and emotions. Change in one domain causes change in the other. MimiLift Facial MuscleCare releases facial tension. This causes overall relaxation, which has important physiological and psychological benefits.

MimiLift is a therapeutic programme based on medical science, which makes it suitable for the rehabilitation of the nerve-muscle functions of the mimic muscles – for example, in cases such as Bell's palsy.

Natural pain relief

MimiLift relieves muscle tension, stiffness and spasms in the face, head and neck. When the muscles relax, the pain decreases. MimiLift alleviates the symptoms of myofascial face and jaw pain and headache. Tension-type headache is a headache of muscular origin that causes pain in the temples, forehead and back of the skull, and it is described as a feeling of tightness or compression in the head. Massage of the aching areas relieves the tension.

MimiLift techniques relieve pain by releasing the body's own, natural chemical modulators of pain, such as endorphins, which are endogenous opioid substances synthesized by the nerve cells.

Massage of the tensed, sore muscles sends signals to the brain along the same nerves as the pain signals. Pleasant signals of the massage suppress the pain signals, because the mild sensation of cutaneous sensory nerves exerts an inhibitory influence on pain.

MimiLift improves blood and lymph circulation of the face, head and neck. Locally increased blood circulation and lymphatic flow help to remove the accumulation of pain-producing (algogenic) substances such as bradykinin or serotonin that may be responsible for muscle pain in the facial area and head. Improved blood circulation also relieves the muscle-related pain by bringing more oxygen to the tensed, tight, ischemic muscles.

Relaxed voice production

MimiLift Facial MuscleCare is excellent for freeing up the voice for speech production and singing. Correctly functioning muscles that move the lip area, the lower jaw and the tongue promote fluent speech. A relaxed jaw is vital for relaxed speech and singing. Singers often need more jaw-opening mobility than the average value. Singers have reported hitting the high notes with greater ease after they have stretched and relaxed their jaw muscles.

MimiLift tongue exercises remove tightness from the muscles moving the tongue and widen the range of motion of the tongue. A relaxed and mobile tongue promotes both clear articulation and relaxation of the mimic and chewing muscles.

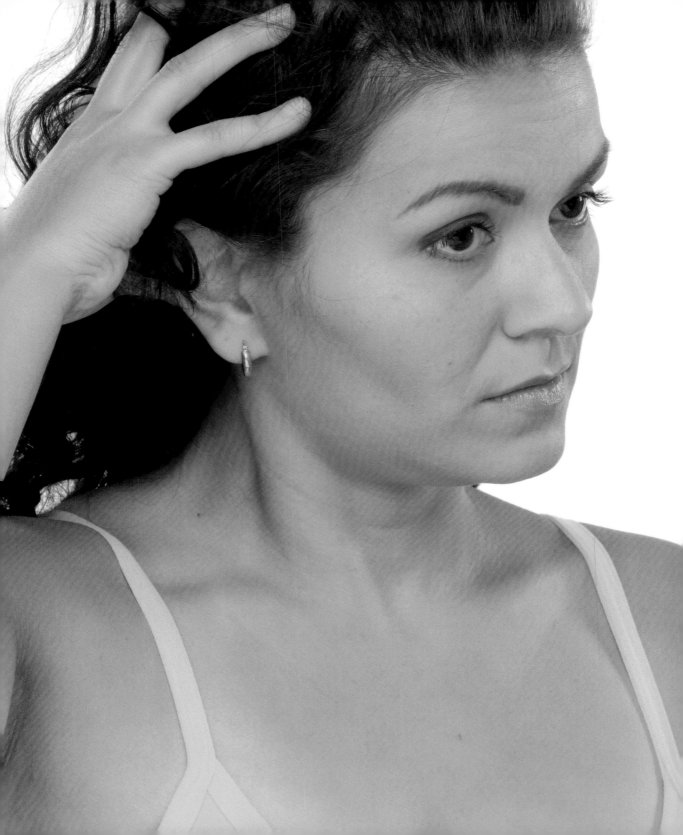

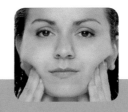

MUSCLES OF THE HEAD

6

RELAXING **THE EYES**

Staring all day at a computer, reading or watching TV for hours, driving a car or any other prolonged visually intensive tasks can strain your eyes. Eye strain is basically the strain of the eye muscles, and it can lead to various problems such as tired, sore eyes and headache. Ergonomic solutions and eye-relaxing procedures will relieve and prevent stress on your eyes.

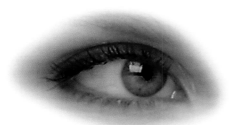 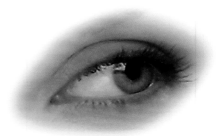

Relax and tone the eye-moving muscles

Six muscles that move the eyeball, the extraocular muscles, are located inside the eye socket and around the eyeball. They are highly innervated voluntary, skeletal muscles. Extraocular muscles of both eyes work smoothly together in a coordinated way to enable both eyes to focus on the same object.

Extraocular muscles work all day long and do not easily show signs of fatigue. However, static overloading muscle work such as staring at the computer can eventually strain the eye muscles. Extraocular muscles can also degenerate with age just like other skeletal muscles.

In order both to relieve tension in all the extraocular muscles and to strengthen them you need to perform precise eye movements in various directions. When the primary muscle that moves the eye in a desired direction is working, the muscle that moves the eye in the opposite direction must relax to allow the movement.

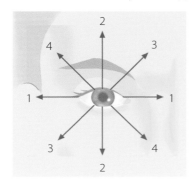

Perform the following eye movements slowly and smoothly, without moving your head. Look in each direction for 2 seconds. Blink normally. Close your eyes for a while at the end of this eye session.

1 look to the right – look to the left
2 look straight up – look straight down
3 look up and to the right – look down and to the left
4 look up and to the left – look down and to the right

Relax the eye-opening muscles

The muscle that elevates the upper eyelid (levator palpebrae muscle) is located deep in the skin of the upper eyelid. When a person gets tired, the tonus of the eyelid-elevating muscle decreases, and the eyes tend to close. Then it is common to raise the eyebrows to help in keeping the eyes open. Static overuse of the muscle that raises the eyebrows, the frontalis muscle, can cause pain over the forehead and an intermittent or constant headache.

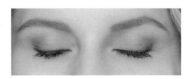

Prevent the eyelid-elevating muscle becoming fatigued by having breaks when you can close your eyes for a minute or two, or rest your eyes completely by taking a nap.

Relax the eye-closing muscles

Habitual squinting for any reason tenses the muscle responsible for this action, the orbicularis oculi muscle. For example, nearsighted people not wearing proper glasses squint to improve their vision to see objects in the distance more clearly.

Chronic tension of the orbicularis oculi muscle may cause local pain above the upper eyelid just below the eyebrow.

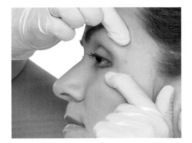

Relieve orbicularis oculi muscle tension with a stretching technique. Stretch the orbicularis oculi muscle by pulling it gently and firmly with fingers in opposite directions.

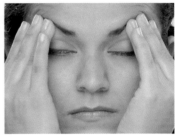

Relieve orbicularis oculi muscle tension with a gliding massage stroke. Slide your fingers right below the eyebrows.

Relax the eye-accommodation muscles

Muscles inside the eye are innervated by the autonomic systems and include the iris sphincter and the ciliary muscle. Darkness makes the iris sphincter dilate the pupils and increased light produces constriction of the pupils. The ciliary muscle is attached to the lens and changes the shape of the lens. For near vision the ciliary muscle contracts and for far vision it relaxes. This process is known as the accommodation of the eye.

Prolonged intensive near use of the eyes such as computer work or reading will strain the ciliary muscle. Viewing an object at a very near distance, under 25 cm, increases eye strain. The human eye is designed to shift focus between near and distant objects, not stare at one point for long periods of time.

When you are at a computer, take a break about every half an hour to divert your eyes from the screen. Shift your focus to at least 6 metres away, by looking out of the window for a minute, for instance.

Prevent dry eyes

The blinking function of the orbicularis oculi muscle spreads tear fluid over the cornea, the transparent front part of the eye. Regular blinking, about 20 times per minute, keeps the eyes from drying out.

Staring too long at a computer screen often reduces the blink rate. The lower blink rate decreases tear production and causes eye moisture to evaporate, resulting in dry, irritated eyes. To avoid the dry eye condition, remind yourself to the blink your eyes regularly.

Check out ergonomics

Check out the ergonomics of your work environment to prevent eye strain. Adjust the screen height and distance, and brightness and contrast on the monitor for the best comfort. Position the computer screen in order to avoid glare and use non-reflective interfaces. Place the monitor so that your line of sight is about 15 degrees below the horizontal line. When possible, read from paper instead of a computer screen.

Check out the environmental factors that may dry your eyes. Keep the air around you humid and use a humidifier if necessary. Avoid draughts from air-conditioning units.

CONTACT A MEDICAL PROFESSIONAL

If you have difficulties in seeing clearly, check with an eye care professional to see if you should wear glasses. People who can see close objects clearly but objects farther away appear blurred are nearsighted. For farsighted people distant objects are clear but close objects are blurred. A common symptom of nearsightedness and farsightedness is eye strain and a headache. If you are already wearing prescription glasses, have an eye examination every two years to make sure your visual acuity is the best it can be.

Changes in vision such as blurriness, blind spots, double vision and dimness of vision should always be evaluated by an ophthalmologist, a medical doctor who is specialized in eye and vision care. When an eye problem is a part of a general health problem, it is treated by a physician specializing in another medical area.

VISION THERAPY

 If the extraocular muscles do not work together, one eye looks at one object and the other eye turns in a different direction. This kind of extraocular imbalance is called strabismus, a condition known as 'crossed eyes'. The brain may learn to ignore the image from the weaker eye, and the vision of the weaker, 'lazier' eye will eventually deteriorate.

In children with strabismus, the problem can usually be corrected with early diagnosis and treatment. The first step in treatment is special glasses or a patch placed over the better eye, which forces the weaker eye to work. Adults with mild strabismus may cope well with glasses and therapeutic eye muscle exercises to keep the eye straight.

Orthoptics is a technique for training the extraocular muscles in order to straighten the misaligned eyes. Orthoptics is a part of a broader range of techniques used to treat a wider variety of vision problems. Vision therapy is prescribed by an optometrist, a health care professional licensed to provide eye care services.

Vision therapy has nothing to do with the non-medical 'throw away your glasses' programmes. Some non-medical programmes include exercises without a proper physiological reason and can cause discomfort, such as the advice to rotate your eyes or to stare at the tip your nose.

RELAXING **SCALP MASSAGE**

The scalp is the part of the head that is usually covered with hair. When the scalp muscles or neck muscles attached to the head become tense, a sensation of tightness around the head can occur, often leading to a headache. Scalp massage relieves tension and gives an overall feeling of relaxation.

Muscles of the scalp

Under the skin of the scalp exists a layer of thin muscles. On the side of the head lies the temporalis muscle, a broad, fan-shaped chewing muscle involved in the closing of the jaw. The back of the head is covered by the occipitalis muscle. There are no muscles on the top of the head, but a flat tendon-like sheet connects the muscle of the forehead, the frontalis muscle, and the muscle of the back of the head, the occipitalis muscle. These two muscles together move the scalp and elevate the eyebrows. Attachments and fascias of the neck muscles that move the head also continue to the area of the scalp.

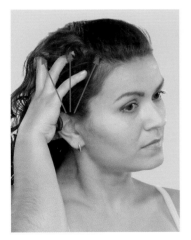

Friction and gliding strokes

1 Spread your fingers slightly and place your fingertips on your scalp. Move your scalp with firm circular movements. Work all over your scalp with this friction stroke. Then keep your fingers spread out and glide your fingers slowly and firmly through your scalp, especially over your temples.

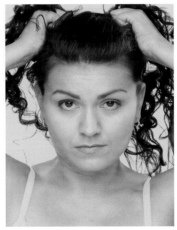

Hair pulling

2 If your hair is long enough, grip a handful of hair near the roots and pull it. Keep on pulling and try to move the scalp gently and rhythmically with tiny up-and-down, back-and-forth or circular movements. Use one hand or both hands, pulling your hair from place to place all over your scalp, a few seconds per position.

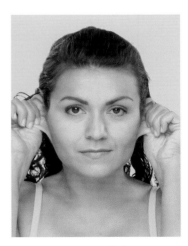

Massage around the ears

3 Grip your ears with your thumbs behind the auricles and other fingers in the front. Lightly pull, vibrate and rub the auricles for a few seconds to get them warm. Then rub a few times around your ears until the feeling of warmth is achieved.

TONGUE EXERCISES

The tongue is made of muscles. The tongue is very movable and its movements are needed for eating and speaking. Tension of the tongue can increase tension in the other nearby muscles, as in the chewing muscles. A proper resting position of the tongue and tongue exercises will reduce extra tension.

The tongue's anatomy and function

The tongue is a solid mass of voluntary, skeletal muscle fibres covered by a mucosal coat. The tongue has two sets of muscles, situated within the tongue and outside it.

The tongue's intrinsic muscles have no attachments to any bones. They alter the shape of the tongue. The tongue's extrinsic muscles are attached to the floor of the mouth, the hyoid bone and the lower jawbone. They move the tongue up and down, from side to side and in and out.

The movements of the tongue are important for eating, swallowing and speaking. The tongue guides the food in the mouth and the movements of the tongue are vital for speech. The tongue is not only a muscular organ, it is also the principal organ for taste.

The tongue's resting position

First check the resting position of your lower jawbone in the upright posture. The space between your upper and lower teeth should be between 2 and 5 mm. In this resting position the tension of the chewing muscles is reduced to a minimum.

After putting your jaw in a proper relaxed position, check the resting position of your tongue. The correct resting position means the position where you are not using your tongue for speaking, eating or swallowing. In the resting position your tongue feels most relaxed. The tip of your tongue should be resting just behind the middle of your front teeth, without pushing the teeth.

In the resting position do not press your tongue against your teeth or against the roof or to the floor of your mouth. These unnecessary habits can easily lead to increased tension in the chewing muscles.

Tongue exercises

IMPACT ON HEALTH: Tongue exercises remove tightness and tension from the muscles moving the tongue and maintain and widen, if necessary, the range of motion of the tongue. A relaxed and mobile tongue promotes clear articulation and fluent speech production. The act of stretching your tongue out relaxes also your chewing muscles.

INSTRUCTIONS

It would be better to wash your face before and after the tongue exercises. These exercises can be performed while taking a shower. Perform the tongue exercises peacefully and slowly in the widest range of motion. Keep your tongue for a while in the maximum position and feel the stretch. Repeat every exercise about 4 times.

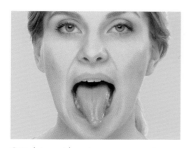

Sticking the tongue out

1 Stick your tongue out straight forward and as far as possible.

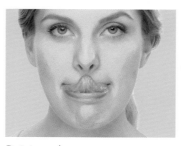

Raising the tongue

2 Raise the tip of your tongue towards your nose. If there is any tightness as you move your tongue in this direction, increase the effectiveness of the exercise by raising your tongue a bit more with your fingers underneath the tongue. You may use a towel between your fingers and your tongue.

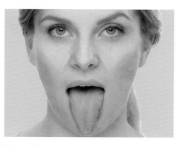

Reaching downward with the tongue

3 Push your tongue downward towards the tip of your chin.

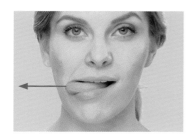

Moving the tongue sideways

4 Reach with your tongue straight to side, towards the cheek. Do the same to the other side.

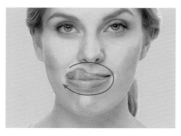

Tongue's circle

5 Stick your tongue out and move it in a large circle, alternating clockwise and counterclockwise.

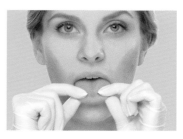

Stretching the intrinsic muscles of the tongue

6 First stick your tongue out. Grasp your tongue with your fingers. Spread the tongue carefully and gently. Use gloves or a towel to prevent the grip slipping.

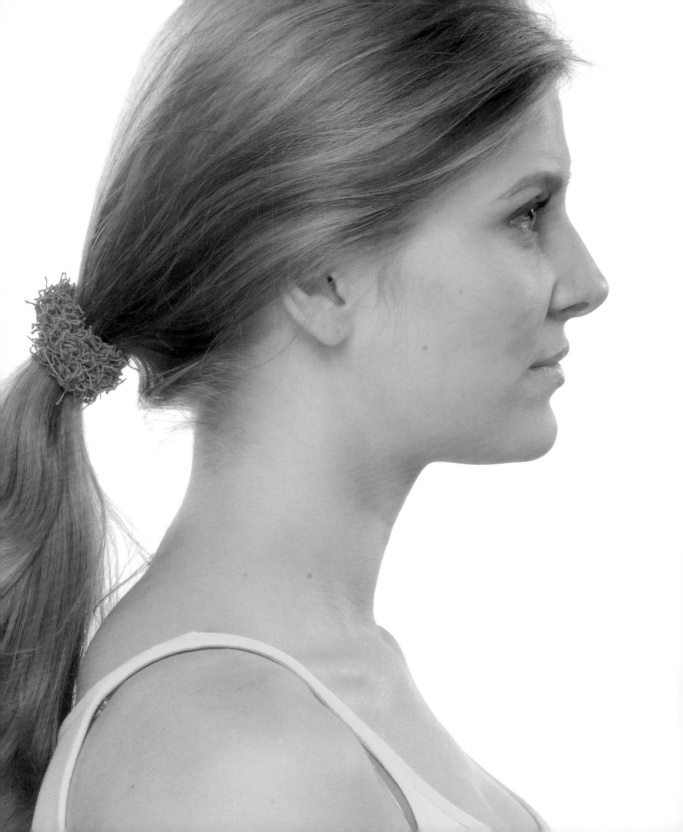

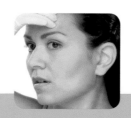

POSTURE
CORRECTION 7

UPPER BODY POSTURE

A forward head posture held for long periods of time may cause pain in the neck-shoulder, head and facial regions. A correct posture prevents muscle tightness and joint overloading, thus contributing to the welfare of the whole musculoskeletal system of the upper body.

Slumped upper body posture

A forward head posture with slumped chest is a common postural problem, especially in people who work at a computer.

IMPACT ON HEALTH: A poor, slumped upper body posture with the head in a forward position causes muscular, ligamentous and disc strain upon the neck, shoulders and the lower back, especially if the posture is maintained for long periods of time and aggravated by the intensity of the work. The muscles of the chest and in the front of the neck become shorter, the muscles of the back and side of the neck become tense and tight and the muscles between the shoulder blades become fatigued and weak.

The shortened, tight muscles in the neck and chest can compress the nerves and blood vessels that supply the arms and hands, leading to symptoms such as a prickling sensation, pain, weakness and coldness in the arms, hands or fingers.

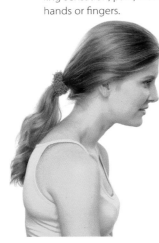

Head and neck forward posture draws the lower jaw backwards which has negative effects on the chewing muscles, jaw joints, rest position of the lower jaw and the bite.

COLLAPSED UPPER BODY POSTURE

- head and neck pushed forward
- altered curvature of the neck
- collapsed chest
- rounded upper back
- shoulders turned forward and inward
- winging shoulders blades

Tension in the chewing muscles increases, the teeth contact will get disturbed and jaw joints will be misloaded.

IMPACT ON APPEARANCE: The slumped posture looks bad, makes a person look tired and much older than he or she actually is. This kind of posture creates also a "neck hump", because when the head and neck are jutted forward, the base of the neck in the upper back looks somewhat humped. The natural spinal curves are altered in the junction where the lowest neck vertebra connects with the uppermost thoracic vertebra, and instead of the normal slight rise, a bigger hump will gradually develop.

Posture is a choice

Posture is in most cases nothing but a learned habit, a good or bad one. A person's feelings and image of his or her own posture is not always the same as it really looks. Someone may consider his or her posture properly erect and lifted, even though in reality it is so slumped that it makes the person a few centimetres shorter than his or her real height would be.

If faulty posture is not a result of disease affecting the joints or the muscles, posture can be improved. In fact, most people can correct their posture quite a lot just in a few seconds, when they are asked to do it. Unfortunately, after few minutes, or even after a few seconds, the old, familiar, bad posture has often returned.

Over the years the person has accepted the slumped and head-forward posture to feel like his or her normal posture. Optimal posture no longer feels normal any longer, because it is so far away from the habitual bad posture.

Correcting posture requires a lot of work at first, mainly becoming aware of the difference between bad and good posture. For the first weeks, the person needs to control his or her posture in all daily activities, and correct the postural alignments many times a day. Eventually, the body will accept the new, better postural habits to be normal.

Good posture

In a balanced posture the body parts, head, chest and pelvis are placed in equilibrium in relation to each other and in relation to the centre of gravity. Good posture places minimal strain on the muscles, ligaments and joints. When the bones and joints are aligned correctly, the muscles work in conjunction with one another with minimum effort. Good posture is comfortable and effortless. It promotes the healthy functioning of the jaw joints and chewing muscles. Good posture simply feels good and looks good.

Good posture is not an uptight military posture. Do not tense your muscles. Do not vigorously push your chest out. Do not pull your abdomen in.

Do not forcibly pull your shoulders back. Maintain an erect posture without unnnecessary forcing or tensing of any of your muscles. Use only as much muscular effort as necessary to correct your postural alignment.

If it is difficult for you to find a suitable posture, ask a physiotherapist with experience of postural re-education to guide your postural aligment. Professional verbal, visual and facilitated guidance can maximize the postural correction efficiently.

POSTURAL EXERCISE

This exercise takes only a minute or two and can be done frequently during the day. It is a break from the sustained slumped postures of many daily activities.

1 Stand with your feet hip-width apart. Feel the crown of your head pulling you up while your feet have solid contact with the ground. Your chest is lifted in a relaxed manner. Your spine is long and extended, yet retaining its natural inward and outward curves. Feel the contact between your feet and the ground. Feel your body's weight drop through the feet. Keep your knees and hips relaxed.

2 Hold the good posture. Turn out your shoulders and the palms of your hands. After reaching this position push your hands gently downwards and slowly move your neck in all directions. Stay for a moment in positions where the muscles of your neck feel tight and feel a relaxing stretch in different parts of your neck. At the end of this postural exercise relax your shoulders and arms, and maintain the good upper body posture.

Posture correction

- On an in-breath, lift your chest, then breathe out and let your chest stay gently lifted, wide and free.
- Let your head go upward.
- Pull the back of your neck up.
- Allow your neck to be free.
- Your head is light and free, delicately balanced on the upper spine.
- Keep your jaw relaxed.
- Keep your chin at horizontal level.
- Relax your shoulders and keep them down.
- Keep your upper back wide by imagining that your shoulders are going away from each other.

TIGHTENING OF **THE NECK MUSCLES**

A balanced action of the neck and head muscles supports proper head position and correct upper body posture. Tightening of any of these muscles will affect the whole system, because the body is a series of musclular, fascial and nervous connections. Tightness and pain in the neck-shoulder region spread easily to the head region and vice versa.

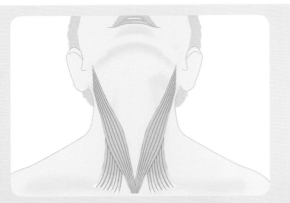

Sternocleidomastoid muscle runs from behind the ears to the collar bones and breast bone. Tightening of this muscle can cause referred pain upwards to the cheek and over the eye, dizziness and tinnitus.

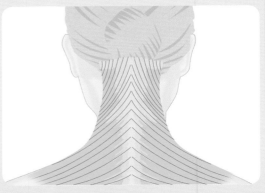

Upper trapezius muscle extends from the base of the skull downwards towards the shoulders. When tight, it may cause referred pain to the side of the head.

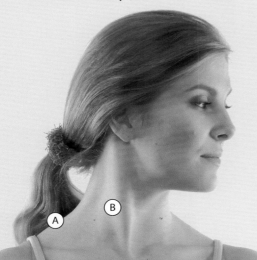

DEEP AND SUPERFICIAL MUSCLES

The skeletal muscles of the body are located in layers. Superficial muscles are just beneath the skin and deep muscles underneath them, closest to the bones. For example, the trapezius muscle (A) and sternocleidomastoid muscle (B) lie in the superficial layer.

Stiff neck affects the jaw

Bad posture strains and tenses the muscles. Sustained muscle tension and tightness compress the blood vessels, leading to reduced blood flow into the muscles involved. Ischemia and accumulation of metabolic waste products result in pain, which causes further tension.

Muscles in the front, side and back of the head that are attached to the skull move the head and play a big part in positioning the head. Head posture affects the position of the lower jawbone. For example, a forward head posture may cause a harmful change in the position of the lower jaw and strain the chewing muscles and jaw joints.

In the long term slumped upper body posture may gradually lead to tension, tightness and pain in the neck-shoulder region. Soreness and tension in this region spread easily into the head and facial area.

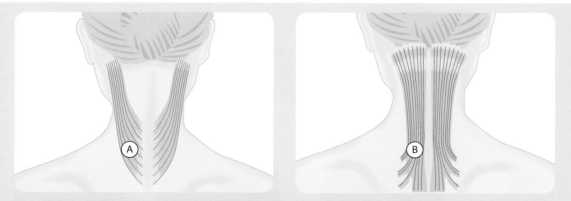

The **splenius capitis muscle** (A) and **semispinalis capitis muscle** (B) connect the back of the skull to several vertebrae of the upper spine. These muscles are involved in headache pains when tightened and tensed.

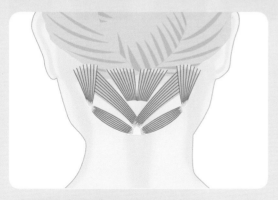

Suboccipital muscles are tiny muscles just underneath the base of the skull. Tightening of these muscles may cause a headache.

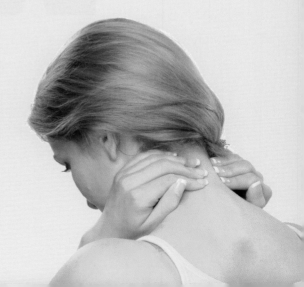

NECK PROGRAMME

The muscles and joints of the neck require motion to stay healthy. Neck movement and stretching exercises and self-massage improve the wellbeing and appearance of the neck-shoulder region and promote a good upper body posture.

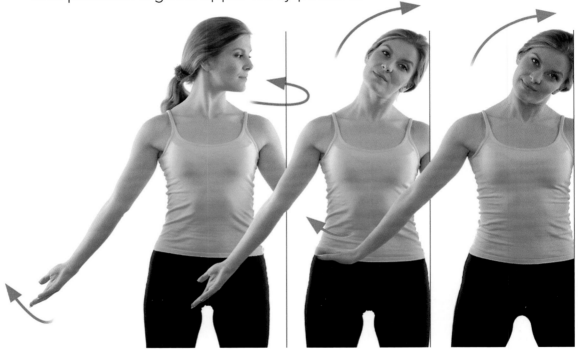

Dynamic neck stretches

1 Elevate your chest and rotate your shoulders and arms outwards. Turn your head gently to both sides as far as it will go without causing any pain.

Keep for a moment near the fullest range of motion available. Perform a pure rotation movement without any side bending.

2 From the same starting position tilt your head slowly from side to side, as if attempting to touch your ear to your shoulder.

Hold your neck for a while in the sideways-bent position and pull your shoulders down. Feel the stretch in the side of your neck.

3 Push your hands downward, flex your wrists and extend your fingers. Incline your head softly, slowly and carefully, alternating directions from straight side to the side, to slightly diagonally upwards and then to diagonally downwards.

Stay in the tightest position for a moment. The feeling of the stretch continues from your neck even to your fingers.

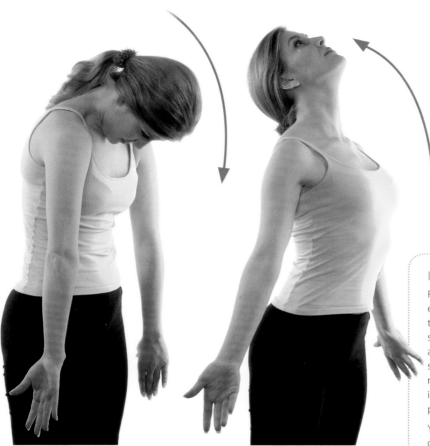

4a Rotate your shoulders and arms inwards, round your upper back and bend your head and neck down to bring your chin towards your chest.

Reach your hands down and feel the stretch in the back of your neck and in your upper back.

4b Make a counter-move by lifting your chest up, by rotating your shoulders and arms outwards and by gently bending your head backwards, as if you were looking up to the sky. This movement should create a slight backwards bending both in your neck and upper back.

Push your hands downward and feel the stretch in the front of your neck and upper chest. Continue by alternating the movements a and b.

INSTRUCTIONS

Repeat every stretching exercise a few times and hold the stretch positions for few seconds. This programme is an excellent exercise break for sedentary workers. Regular neck movement and stretching exercises will loosen and prevent stiffness in the neck.

You may hear creaks, crackles or crunches as you move your neck. They are natural noises coming from the structures of your neck and are nothing to worry about.

Anyone with a cervical spine instability due to rheumatoid arthritis, a trapped nerve in the neck, a cervical disc prolapse or other serious neck condition should consult their treating physician before attempting any neck exercises.

Thoracic spine mobilization

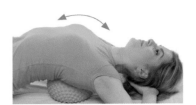

Lie down over a ball with a diameter of approximately 18 cm. Support your head with your hands or with a thin pillow. At first place the ball between your shoulder blades, then change the place of the ball between slightly up and down. However, the ball should remain under the thoracic spine.

Relax for a while in every position. Breathe deeply and try to extend your arms gently over your head, back of the hands near the floor.

If you do not have a ball, you can use sheets wrapped into a tight roll.

This passive backward-bending is a therapeutic exercise after leaning over a computer for many hours. It improves the mobility of the thoracic spine and the ribs and is a good counter-move for a slumped upper body posture.

Relaxing the upper neck and the back of the head

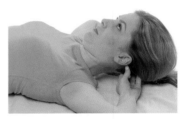

Lie on your back. Place your fingers against the back of your skull. Keep your neck relaxed and let your hands support the weight of your head.

Apply firm, calm circular pressures with the fingers of both hands throughout the base of the skull. Keep your chin down and your eyes closed. Let your head follow the movements softly. Concentrate on relaxing the muscles of your upper neck, and let the feeling of relaxation spread all over your head.

Static neck stretches

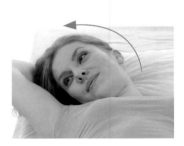

Lie on your back, with your head on a thin pillow or a folded towel. The shoulder of the side of the stretch is lowered and the hand is extended downwards or anchored under the buttock. The opposite hand reaches near the ear and takes a solid grip of the head.

With the help of the hand, slowly, carefully and softly pull your head and neck into side-bending, face looking forwards. Then change the stretch with small variations, by turning your head a little toward the direction of pull and then away from it. Keep your shoulder down and against the cushion. Varying degrees of neck flexion and rotation can be used to direct the stretch to different areas in the neck.

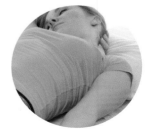

Hold every stretch for a few seconds. Concentrate on the feelings of the stretches, and choose the directions in which the muscles in the side, in the back and in the front of your neck feel tightest.

Return your head slowly to the mid-position and do the same stretches to the other side.

SELF-MASSAGE OF THE NECK

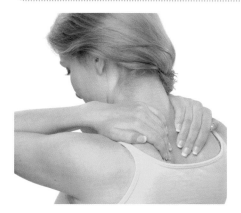
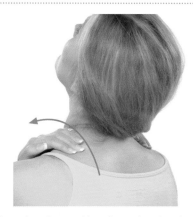

1 Put your hands over your shoulders, near your upper thoracic spine, and bend your head and neck down. Draw your hands across your shoulders towards your collar bones with a strong gliding stroke, and raise your head up at the same time.

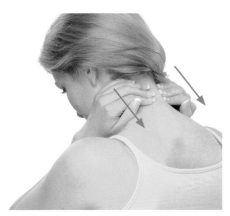
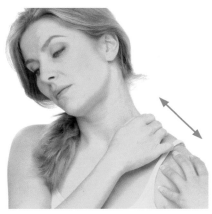

2 Place your fingers at the back of your neck on either side of the cervical spine. Let your head drop forward. At first glide firmly and evenly along the muscles in the back of your neck, the stroke proceeding from the base of the skull towards the shoulders. Then carefully apply firm circular pressures, working down your neck.

3 In order to remove muscle knots in your neck and shoulder region, apply small back-and-forth movements in the direction of the muscle fibres. Use the opposite hand to massage, and keep your head tilted to the other side during the massage. Increase the pressure where you feel most tight. Massage both sides.

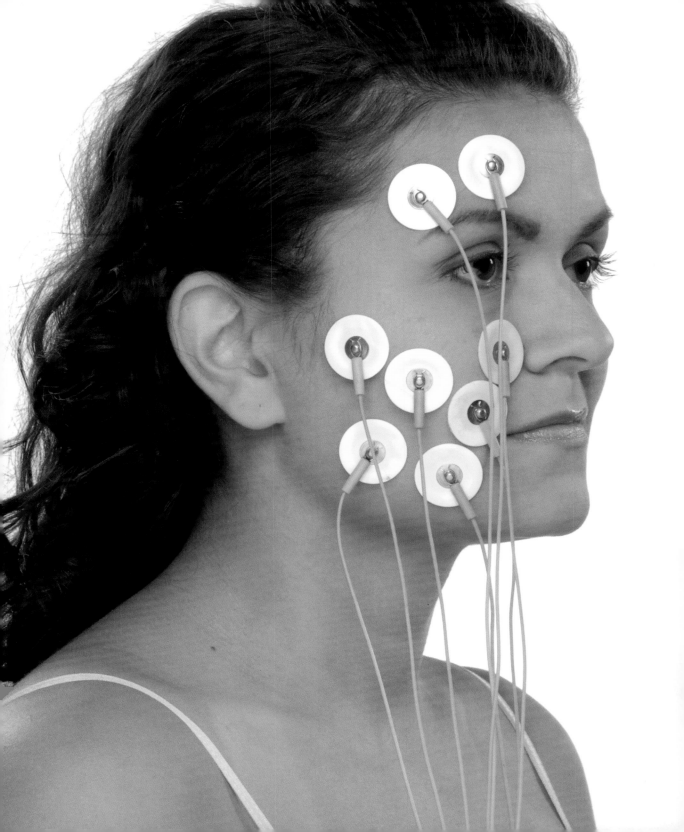

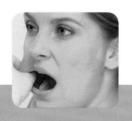

SUPPORTIVE
SELF-TREATMENTS 8

HEAT AND COLD THERAPY

Moist heat packs can be used for self-treating chronic muscle-based pains of the face. They work best in combination with other treatments, massage and stretching. Cold packs are used to treat acute pain, swelling and inflammation.

Heat therapy

Topical heat packs transfer heat to the tissues. Heat therapy is mainly used for chronic conditions. Facial heat therapy increases regional blood flow both in the skin and in the muscles, relaxes tensed facial musculature, eases chronic muscle-based facial pain and temporarily decreases stiffness of the soft tissues.

Heat packs provide a relaxing pre-treatment for very tight and tensed chewing muscles before massaging or stretching them. Heat therapy in the form of a facial steam bath impacts both on facial health and appearance. In addition to soothing tensed facial musculature, it gives the face a healthy colour and glow.

PROCEDURE: Commercially available reusable **heat gel packs** stay warm long enough to produce an effective heat treatment. Warm the pack in hot water, wrap the heated pack in a warm moist towel, and apply the pack to the chewing muscles, the masseter and temporalis muscles. You don't have to press the pack with your hands, if you put a wide band or scarf from under your chin, over your ears to the top of your head and place the hot packs under it against your chewing muscles.

> **LOCAL EFFECTS OF HEAT THERAPY**
>
> - widening of the blood capillary vessels
> - metabolic increase
> - increase in motor and sensory nerve conduction
> - increase in tissue elasticity, collagen extensibility
> - decrease in muscle tone

You can also use a **hot water bottle** wrapped inside a moist piece of cloth or simply a **moist warm towel** or wool cloth which is soaked in hot water and then spun dried. Because the towels cool quite rapidly, you have to wet them in hot water every five minutes or so.

Before applying the heat compress to the face, test the compress by touching it with your fingers to make sure it is not too hot. Very high temperatures may cause burning. If the hot pack becomes uncomfortable during the treatment, remove it.

Heat pack treatment lasts from 20 to 30 minutes. You can repeat the heat therapy a few times a day, if needed. The procedure is most comfortable if you lie down, close your eyes and enjoy the relaxing feeling of the warmth.

A homemade **facial steam bath** is created by pouring boiling water into a bowl and leaning the face over it. Cover your head and upper body with a thick towel. Stay under the steam for a few minutes. Make sure that your face maintains a safe distance from the water. You may add herbs or a few drops of aromatherapy oil to the

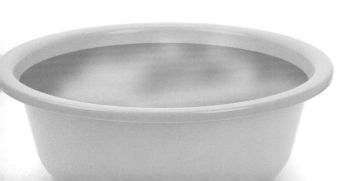

water to give extra pleasure through the wonderful scent. A facial steam bath is a handy way to refresh and invigorate the face whenever it looks tired and stressed. If your face feels tight in the morning just after waking up, the hot steam helps to relax the tensed facial musculature quickly.

CAUTION: Do not use heat therapy on tissues with acute trauma or infections, because in these cases heat worsens the symptoms and slows down the healing process. Heat packs cannot be used to treat people with impaired sensations because insensitive skin would be at risk of burning.

Cold therapy

Topically applied cold packs withdraw the warmth from the tissues. Cold therapy is generally used in acute traumatic and inflammatory conditions, such as immediately after a blow to the face or in acute jaw joint pain. Cold therapy is recommended especially for the first two days following an injury.

The application of cold is beneficial for reducing the inflammatory processes by slowing down the flow of blood and other fluids to the injured area. Consequently, this reduces the swelling and bruising, and speeds up the healing process. Compressing a sore point with cold eases the pain. Cold numbs the nerves, which reduces the pain sensations.

PROCEDURE: Cold packs include home-made **ice bags**, commercial resusable gel packs and disposable chemical packs. For an ice bag, place several ice cubes in a plastic bag, close it tightly with a knot, wrap in a towel and crush the cubes with a hammer. A **reusable gel pack** becomes cold in a freezer in two hours or it can be stored in the freezer between uses. **Disposable chemical packs** becomes cold by squeezing the pack firmly.

Before applying the cold pack to the area to be treated, wrap it in a cold, moist, thin towel. The cloth provides a barrier to eliminate frostbite and reduces the discomfort associated with the cold pack's initial contact with the skin. Apply the cold pack to the desired area of the

> **LOCAL EFFECTS OF COLD THERAPY**
>
> - constriction of the blood capillary vessels
> - metabolic decrease
> - decrease in motor and sensory nerve conduction
> - decrease in tissue elasticity

face until the tissue feels numb, but for no longer than about 8 minutes. Remove the pack if it feels uncomfortable. You can repeat the treatment several times, but let the area get slowly warm again before applying another cold pack.

CAUTION: Cold intolerance, impaired sensation and insensitive skin are conditions where cold therapy cannot be used. Nor can cold packs be placed on regenerating peripheral nerves. If a nerve is injured in the periphery, the cold treatment would worsen the nerve's already impaired ability to transmit impulses.

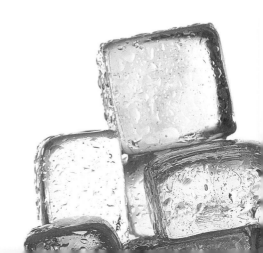

ELECTROTHERAPY

Electrotherapy can be used to enhance both facial beauty and health. The combination of gentle facial electrostimulation and simultaneous voluntary facial muscle work strengthens facial muscles and ligaments effectively for a more lifted appearance. In health care mild specific electrical currents are used to relieve acute and chronic facial pains.

What is electrotherapy?

In electrotherapy gentle electrical currents stimulate a muscle or a nerve, in order to strengthen muscles or to alleviate pain. It is a safe and technologically advanced form of treatment, having been used within the medical field for over 40 years.

Electrotherapy is based on the existence of electricity in most of the cells of the human body. Many functions of the body are controlled by the body's own electrical impulses. For example, when you exercise, natural electrical impulses cause your muscles to contract. The electrotherapy device imitates these impulses, making the muscles contract and relax rhythmically in a pattern similar to normal exercise.

The frequency and intensity of the current and the stimulation time determine the effects of the electrotherapy. Frequency refers to the number of pulses per second and is measured in Hertz. So 50 Hz means a frequency of 50 pulses per second.

Frequencies of 10–70 Hz cause muscle contractions when the stimulation or contraction time is long enough and the intensity is high enough. Frequencies 1–10 Hz and 75–100 Hz are used for pain suppression.

Electrical facial muscle stimulation

The most common – although not the most highly recommended – way to use electrical facial muscle stimulation is simply to let the current contract the facial musculature and create uncontrolled,

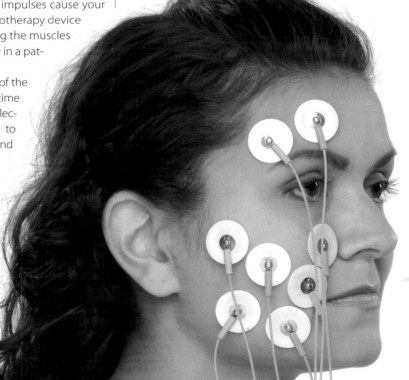

uncoordinated facial movements while the client is passive. Instead, in MimiLift Facial MuscleCare passive electronic muscle stimulation is combined with simultaneous active, cognitive and coordinated facial muscle work. When an electronic signal starts, a simultaneous voluntary facial movement is executed in the same direction as induced by the electrical stimulation.

This kind of functional electrical facial muscle stimulation activates the entire muscle, even the parts of the muscle that are rarely used. It is also the most comfortable way to use electrostimulation, because associating the electrically stimulated contractions with voluntary muscle contractions will diminish any uncomfortable sensations of the current, such as shooting pains in the teeth.

Electrostimulated functional facial training permits more intensive and longer-lasting sessions than a voluntary facial exercise only, offering effects comparable to serious weight training. The face will feel firmer and look filled, lifted and more toned.

Electrotherapy in health care

The rhythmic muscle movements produced by electrical muscle stimulation increase blood and lymphatic circulation and metabolism of the muscles. Greater quantities of oxygen-rich blood are carried to the tissues and waste products are carried away, resulting in pain relief and relaxation in chronically sore and stiff facial muscles. Rhythmic muscle contractions also stimulate the release of the body's own morphine-like substances, which produce an anaesthetizing effect.

One form of electrical stimulation uses currents that do not cause muscle contractions – only a tingling sensation may be felt. The purpose of these currents is pain management. Short signals at low frequency, from 2 to 10 Hz, help to stimulate the release of the natural anaesthetic chemicals such as endorphins, and sustained stimulation has an effect on managing chronic pain. High frequency stimulation, 75 to 150 Hz, interferes with the pain messages at the spinal cord level and helps to block their transmission to the brain. Alternating different frequencies can provide a natural way to relieve pain.

FUNCTIONAL ELECTRICAL FACIAL MUSCLE STIMULATION

Physiological effects

- increases the strength of facial muscles and ligaments
- increases blood circulation in facial muscles and skin
- increases facial lymphatic flow
- stimulates the skin's fibroblast cells to produce new collagen, elastin and ground substance

Impacts on appearance

- increases and helps to maintain the volume of the facial musculature
- lifts facial contours
- prevents facial sagging
- reduces facial puffiness
- improves facial skin tone
- gives face a healthy glow

General instructions for an electrical facelift

1 Before starting to use the electrical facial muscle stimulation become familiar with your facial muscles, their location and the movements they produce. Learn to perform the voluntary facial muscle exercises properly at first.

2 The electrodes must be positioned on the most appropriate facial muscles to create a natural facelift. Position a pair of electrodes on one facial muscle or muscle group working in the same direction, upwards or sideways. Use soft, self-adhesive facial electrodes with a pad diameter of approximately 2.5 cm that fit the different locations of the face.

3 Turn up the intensity dials until a clear, smooth muscle movement is seen and felt. A mild tingling without an evident muscle contraction is not enough. The intensity must be high enough but not painful. There is a limit to the intensity

of contraction, and impulses exceeding the limit only generate pain.

4 Concentrate and pay attention to the electrical stimulus, sense the passive muscle movement caused by the electrical signal and immediately take part in the movement with your own active parallel facial movement.

5 Always contract the muscle at the same time as it is electrically stimulated by the device. Contract the muscles through their full range of motion. Place the pads and set the intensity so that the muscle contraction feels and seems equal in both sides of the face.

6 A good electrostimulated contraction time for facial muscles varies between 3 and 8 seconds. A short pause follows every contraction, allowing the muscles to return to the starting

position and relax. For a stimulator with four outlets you may need to split the electrical facelift into two sessions by changing the place of the electrodes from one area to another and repeating the stimulation.

7 The total time of the session should be at least 20 to 30 minutes, even 45 minutes if you like. In a session of 20 minutes there will be around 160 muscle contractions or repetitions of a facial muscle movement. The session may be spent for example in a half-sitting position while watching TV. Have sessions at first every other day in a period of 6 to 8 weeks, then at least twice a week to keep your face in shape. For the sake of variety and for more isolated facial movements, do the voluntary facial exercises without the commands of the electric coach every now and then.

Electrical stimulation may also be used as a highly specialized medical therapeutic tool to activate muscles affected by impairment resulting from neurological diseases. For example, mild to moderate difficulties in swallowing due to multiple sclerosis or stroke can be helped by electrical stimulation applied through electrodes placed on the front of the neck.

Electrical muscle stimulator devices

The operation principles of the electrotherapy equipments are quite similar. Electrical stimulators have outlets known as channels. Each channel has

MIMILIFT AND ELECTROTHERAPY

The concept of combining functional electrical facial muscle stimulation with the massage and stretching techniques of MimiLift Facial MuscleCare is likely to lead to the most significant results. Strengthening exercises must be balanced with stretching exercises in order to avoid excessive tightening of the facial musculature.

two wire connections with two electrodes attached at the end of each lead wire. The electrical device delivers electronic impulses via soft electrode pads which are applied to the surface of the skin on an area of a particular muscle or muscle group. The impulses generated by the device travel across the skin and flow between the pair of electrodes. The underlying muscle responds by contracting and relaxing rhythmically.

If you are planning to buy an electrical stimulator for individual home use, there are many kind of devices available. Read the manufacturer's information carefully, and do not hesitate to ask for more information from the vendor. Some devices are more suitable for pain management than for electrical muscle stimulation, and devices delivering only microcurrent are completely unable to cause any muscle contractions. Microcurrent is an electrical current of a millionth of an ampere, so low that it is often impossible even to feel it, and so low that it can never cause a muscle to contract.

The simplest machines offer merely a monotonous repetition of a same signal. They have usually only one outlet with one pair of electrodes, in which case you should change their place many times in one session in order to reach many facial areas.

More developed automated units with different sequences of signals produce a variety of patterns of activity. Changing patterns of frequencies, contraction and relaxation timings and intensities provide the most effective treatment for an electrical facelift. The most advanced, sophisticated electrical stimulators have microprocessor-controlled programmes, which automatically vary, cycling through many different settings in each programme. They are hands-free, with preferably 4 outlets.

Make sure your choice of machines has been tested and certified to conform to the high standards for medical electrical equipment. The best microcomputerized units for a facelift have scientifically selected pre-set programmes with varying contraction and relaxation times and pulses per second, specially designed to strengthen facial musculature.

You buy a high-quality electrical stimulator device only once and the only ongoing cost is the inexpensive self-adhesive electrode pads.

CAUTION: Electrical stimulation is suitable for most healthy adults, but should not be used by persons with a cardiac pacemaker or when epilepsy is suspected or diagnosed. If you have any other medical condition that you think may affect your ability to use electrical stimulation, consult your doctor.

Basic electrode placements for an electrical facelift

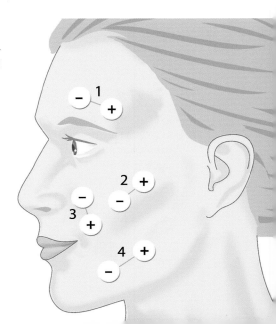

1 **DESIRED MOVEMENT**: Raising of the eyebrows, especially the outer parts of the eyebrows. Regulate the stimulation time of the forehead muscle in order to avoid excessive tensing of the scalp.
GOAL: Lifting of the eyebrows.

2 **DESIRED MOVEMENT:** Pulling the corners of the mouth upwards and elevating the musculature covering the cheekbones.
GOAL: Lifting of the cheeks.

3 **DESIRED MOVEMENT**: Raising the upper lip and the cheek.
GOAL: Lifting of the midface.

4 **DESIRED MOVEMENT:** Drawing the corners of the mouth straight to the side, activating of the jawline.
GOAL: Lifting and reshaping the lower face and lifting the jowls for a defined jawline.

SUPPORTIVE **LIFESTYLE CHOICES**

What matters most for health – genes or lifestyle? For most people it is the cumulative effects of many daily lifestyle choices. A nutrient-rich diet, sleep, exercise and positive emotions are the pillars of a good health and good looks.

Eat well

Your entire body requires proper, balanced nutrition in order to function well and re-generate. Nutritional deficiencies may be one factor behind skin problems, premature ageing or pains attributed to muscles and their surrounding fascias.

Proteins, carbohydrates and fats provide energy for the cells and serve as the building blocks for cellular pro-duction and new tissues. Vitamins and minerals do not contain energy, but have important metabolic roles.

1 **Proteins** from the diet are vital for main-tenance, repair and replenishing of the body's tissues, including the skin and muscles. The daily protein intake should be approximately 0.8–1.8g of protein for every kilogram of the body weight, depending on age and activity level.

Foods that contain high amounts of pro-tein are poultry, red meat, fish, eggs, dairy products, beans (including soy), nuts and seeds. For instance, a 100g serv-ing of chicken contains about 20g of protein and 100g of cheese contains 20–30g of protein.

A lack of protein not only has a harmful effect on skin, but also undermines the person's overall health. Low-protein diets are rec-ommended only for people with certain diseases in which the body cannot metabolize protein, such as kidney disorders.

2 **Essential fatty acids** are important structural components of the cell membranes, and the body needs fats to transport vitamins A, D, E and K around the body. Omega-3 group fats are found in coldwater fish and omega-6 group fats are found in vegatable oils, nuts, seeds and avocados.

Essential fatty acids play an impor-tant role in the healthy function of the brain, skin and eyes. Signs of a deficiency in essential fatty acids include dry skin, increased susceptibility to infection and poor wound healing.

There is no need to follow a fat-free diet. You only need to cut down on the bad fats such as trans fatty acids found in foods containing processed vegetable oils. They are named 'partially hydrogenated vegetable oils' on food labels.

3 **Plant-based foods,** fruits, vegetables, legumes, whole grains and nuts provide essential vitamins and minerals and healthy phytochemicals. For instance, vitamins A and C boost collagen production of the skin, B vitamins are required for normal nervous system function, and calcium and potassium are needed for muscle function.

Plant-based foods have a high capacity of antioxidants – the substances that may protect the cells against the cell-damaging free radicals pro-duced, for example, by excessive UV radiation, heavy consumption of alcohol or smoking.

4 **Multivitamin and mineral supplements** can be useful, but supplements should never used as a substitute for a healthy, varied, nutritious diet. Mega-doses of vitamin or mineral supplements might disrupt the body's biochemical balance. Some of them, such as vitamin A, are toxic in high doses. Choose all-round multivitamin and mineral supplements which include quantities close to the recommended daily allowance of the essential vitamins and minerals.

5 **Water** or fluid is also a vital component of the diet, because about 40–70% of the adult body is comprised of water and requires a proper hydration to stay healthy. Many kind of drinks and water-based foods such as fruits and vegetables are the sources of the fluids in the diet.

There is no evidence that there is any benefit to be gained from drinking increased amounts of water. Let your thirst be your guide. If your urine is slightly yellow, it is a good indication that you are well hydrated. If it is dark yellow, you probably need to drink more.

Alcohol draws water from the body. The body reacts to alcohol like a poison and tries to get rid of it. Part of the process is increased urination and sweating, which make the body lose a great quantity of water and electrolytes. Drinking too much alcohol dehydrates the body internally and also dehydrates the skin, causing it to lose its dewy appearance and making lines and wrinkles more visible. In addition to dehydration, alcohol abuse depletes a person of essential nutrients, particularly A, C and B complex vitamins.

EFFECTS OF SLEEP DEPRIVATION

- Raises the levels of blood glucose, which exposes a person to many diseases such as diabetes and accelerates the ageing process by raising the level of sugars in the tissues.

- Increases the secretion of stress hormones, which may increase muscle tension, heart rate and blood pressure.

- A person not getting enough sleep will lose his or her muscle mass, because the stress hormone cortisol breaks down muscle tissue.

- Decreases the secretion of the body's own anabolic hormones, such as growth hormone.

- Weakens the immune system, so that the ability to fight viral and bacterial diseases deteriorates.

- Impairs brain function, is detrimental to creative thinking and action planning, and changes the mood in a negative direction.

- Increases sensitivity to pain, because the body´s pain system does not have time to recover from the fatigue.

- Impairs motor skills, thus increasing the risk of accidents.

Get enough sleep

The tissues of the body need sleep to recover and renew. Lack of sleep means that the diurnal amount of sleep remains less than the amount that person needs to be energetic in the following day. Even two hours' lack of sleep has a significant impact on health. If you sleep too little for just one week, your condition will decline.

Even a short-term lack of sleep appears on the face. Researches at the Swedish Karolinska Institutet have proved that too little sleep will make a person look less attractive. They conducted an experiment in which they took photos of healthy men and women aged between 18 and 31, both after they had slept enough and after sleep loss.

The pairs of photos were showed to 65 students, who judged that sleep deprivation made the subjects look more tired, less healthy and less attractive. As a well-rested face appears to be attractive, the idea of beauty sleep really does work.

1 **Get a good night's sleep.** The need for sleep is individual. The minimun amount of sleep for most adults is 7.5–9 hours a night. Today, many people sleep only 5–6 hours per night on a regular basis and consider this sleep curtailment harmless.

If you feel tired at any time during the day, this might be the simplest symptom telling that you are not having enough sleep. Listen to your body and sleep longer at nights if necessary.

2 **Take a nap.** A short nap of no more than 15–30 minutes improves alertness and performance. When taking longer naps, the sleeper enters deeper sleep stages and is thus still half-asleep after waking up. The drowsy feeling after a nap of an hour or longer may last up to couple of hours.

3 **A suitable pillow and mattress,** which support the sleeper in a comfortable, ergonomic body position, will promote good-quality sleep. You can find a good position for your whole spine if you sleep lying on your side or on your back. Sleeping on your stomach causes a lot of strain, especially to the cervical spine and the muscles moving it.

The mattress is unsuitable if you wake up in the night because of numbness in parts of your body or if when awakening in the morning your body feels stiff and dull. The pillow is too low if you need to place your hands under the pillow or under your head to support the position of your head.

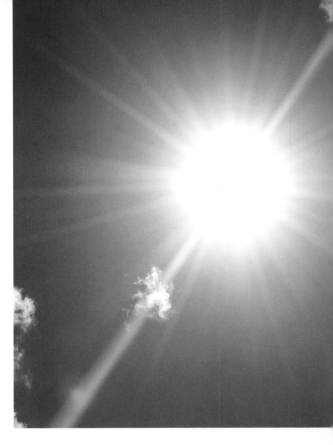

UV protection

Ultraviolet radiation comes naturally from the sun or from manmade lamps. Natural sunlight contains mainly UV-A and shorter-wave UV-B rays. Repeated unprotected exposure to both rays can damage the skin and the eyes, suppress the immune system and raise a person's risk of developing skin cancer. Frequent use of tanning booths and beds is as harmful and dangerous as too much sunlight, because they emit high levels of UV-A.

Overexposure to UV radiation stimulates the production of a collagen-degrading enzyme called collagenase. Normally, small quantities of this enzyme are needed to remove excessive collagen build-up over a healing wound, but when activated by the UV-rays, it will destroy the healthy collagen of the dermis, resulting in the formation of wrinkles.

Many people still regard a tan as a sign of a good health and consider it attractive. Actually, a golden tan is nothing but a sign of a skin damage. A tan means that skin that has been damaged by ultraviolet radiation has increased melanin pigment production for defence purposes.

The intensity of the ultraviolet radiation depends on the location on earth's surface and the time of the year. Small amounts of UV radiation are beneficial, but excessive amounts are harmful. Simple precautions will prevent both short-term and long-term damage ultraviolet radiation, while still making the time spent outdoors enjoyable.

1 **Seek shade** when the sun shines highest overhead and the radiation is therefore the strongest – from about 10 a.m. until 4 p.m. Reflection from the snow, water, sand and even from concrete increases the strength of UV radiation and your risk of overexposure. Cloudy skies do not offer a significant protection from UV rays.

2 **Wear protective clothing.** Ensure that your clothes will screen out UV rays by placing your hand inside the garments and checking that you can't see it through them. A broad-brimmed hat will protect your face.

3 **Use a sunscreen** with SPF (Sun Protection Factor) 30 or higher. Apply it generously and reapply as recommended on the label of the product. Choose a sunscreen that provides both UV-A and UV-B protection. Sunscreens contain chemical UV filters or mainly zinc oxide or titanium oxide which block out the sun rays by forming a physical barrier.

The SPF in the sunscreen filters the ultraviolet rays, but no sunscreen can provide 100% protection from the sun and no sunscreen can completely prevent sunburn, photoageing or skin cancer. Sunscreens provide better protection against UV-B rays than UV-A rays, leaving the skin vulnerable to premature ageing.

4 **Wear sunglasses** to protect your eyes from a very bright sunlight. Do not simply use darkened lenses. Purchase sunglasses with special UV-filters, with labels ensuring that they provide 100% UV protection.

Happiness promotes health

Anger and hostility make a person age more quickly. Researchers from Harvard University studied the effects of anger on health of 670 men taking part in an eight-year ageing survey. They found that the chronically angry men aged prematurely.

Long-lasting high levels of anger and hostility have many harmful effects on the body. Those unable to control their anger are more likely to suffer from headaches, digestion problems, high blood pressure and heart disease.

People who are unable to control their anger damage not only themselves, but also those around them, because hostility communicates fast and automatically from an angry person to other people through facial and vocal expressions.

Laugh the stress away. A study published from Loma Linda University (Berk, *et al.* 1989) has shown that laughter and even simply anticipating a laugh has effective therapeutic effects. Laughing lowers blood pressure, decreases stress hormone levels, relaxes muscles, activates the immune system, releases the body's natural painkillers and creates a general feeling of mental and physical wellbeing.

Seek positive, happy and joyful situations when making choices regarding reading, TV viewing, listening to music or social events. Spend time with friends who make you laugh.

A good hearty laugh is also beneficial for the appearance, because laughing and smiling strengthen the cheek muscles that give the face a lift. A smiling face is also generally considered more attractive and younger than a face with a negative expression.

Daily choices affect long-term happiness. According to the results of a 25-year study of 60,000 people, researchers of the University of Melbourne (Headey, Muffels, Wagner 2010) found that people who prioritized altruistic behaviour, family, friends, social activities, exercise and working the right amount were rewarded with a long-term increase in life satisfaction. Those who prioritized career and material success experienced a corresponding lasting decline.

MOVE YOUR BODY

Regular physical activity, preferably every other day or even more often, is essential for optimal health and has remarkable physiological and psychological benefits. For instance, when you exercise, your body flushes away stress hormones, releases feel-good chemicals called endorphins, and excess tension in your muscles reduces.

Choose an activity you enjoy, walking, swimming, dancing – any form of exercise you like and can make a part of your regular routine. Exercise triggers positive effects both in your body and mind.

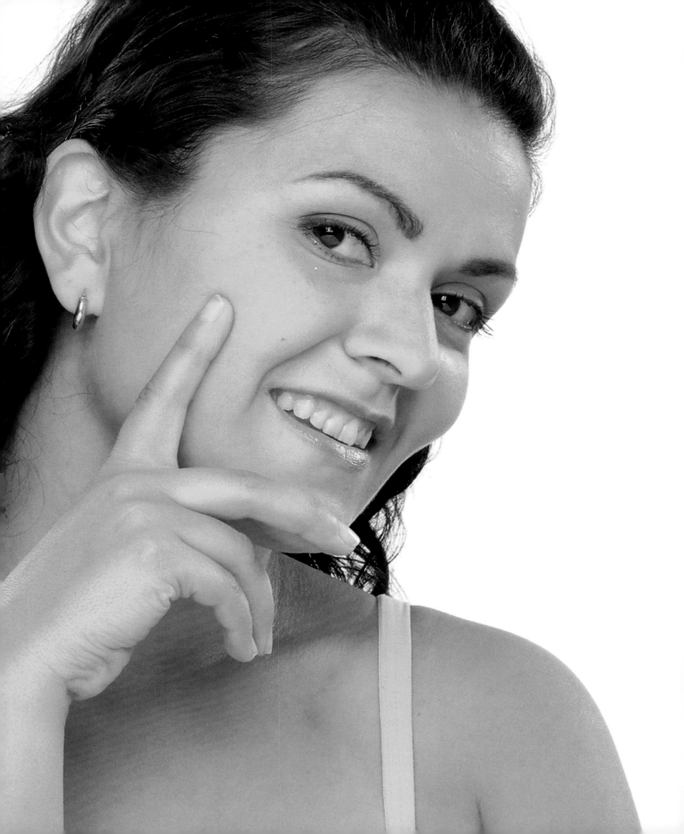

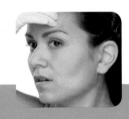

MIMILIFT NATURAL FACIAL
REJUVENATION **9**

MIMILIFT **NATURAL FACELIFTING**

MimiLift Facial MuscleCare improves the condition of the facial muscles and strengthens their attachments to the facial bones. Besides being stronger, fuller, firmer and more elastic than weaker muscles, well-toned facial musculature is better able to resist the sagging of facial features.

Use it or lose it

Facial muscles benefit from strengthening exercises just like other skeletal muscles. Well-toned muscles give a defined shape to both the face and the rest of the body. If unused, however, all voluntary muscles atrophy easily. The reason why facial muscles gradually lose their tone, strength and size is because they are seldom asked to perform varied effective movements in the full range of motion available to them.

As a consequence, muscle cells in the facial muscles become smaller and the supporting ligaments and fascias weaken. The face loses part of its volume, facial musculature becomes flabby and facial features begin to sag. This results in droopy eyebrows and eyelids, sagging cheeks and the shape of the face turning more squarish in shape because tissues around the jawline start to sag.

These changes in our appearance are not a direct result of how old we are, but are partly due to our genes and largely to the way we have used our facial muscles and the cumulative effects of lifestyle factors.

MimiLift face gym

In order to function well and remain strong, firm and shapely, muscles need to be subjected to physical load on a regular basis. Muscle-strengthening exercises can be done at any age. Muscles of the body can be easily strengthened by working out with weights, and MimiLift Facial MuscleCare exercises do the same for the facial muscles.

MimiLift facelifting procedures address the mimic muscles of the face that contribute to the lifting of facial features. The strengthening exercises challenge the muscles to perform the movements in the widest possible range of motion available to them. This means that increasingly more motor units in the facial muscles are recruited, which in turn builds up the proportion of active muscle tissue. With the number of action and myosin filaments in the muscles increasing, muscle cells grow in size and facial muscles become stronger. At the same time MimiLift procedures strengthen the fascial attachments and ligamentous support. Furthermore, with exercise, blood capillaries in the facial muscle tissue dilate, which permits increased blood flow and supply of oxygen and nutrients to facial muscles.

These are some of the ways in which MimiLift Facial MuscleCare improves the condition and function of the facial muscles. Well-conditioned facial muscles have increased body, elasticity and firmness, enabling them to add volume to the face and, together with better ligamentous support, to resist the sagging of facial features.

MIMILIFT **NATURAL LINE SMOOTHING**

The relaxing procedures of MimiLift remove tightness from the mimic muscles and smooth out fine lines and creases. Relaxed facial muscles make facial features soft and give the face a peaceful, pleasant look.

Tightening habits

Tight skeletal muscles impact our posture, while tight mimic muscles result in lines in the face. The unfavourable impact of muscle tightness on the body and face can be addressed by a good stretching and massage routine.

Long-term, continuous strain on muscles makes them taut and short. Working at the computer with the head pushed forward and shoulders hunched up stiffens muscles in the neck and shoulders. Poor postural habits shorten muscles and are reflected in postural misalignment. In the facial area, over the years, it is certain habitual, prolonged facial expressions that tighten the mimic muscles, causing lines to appear in the skin covering the overactive, taut muscles.

These lines run crosswise to the direction in which muscle cells in the mimic muscles are arranged. For example, habitual frowning tightens the muscles between the eyebrows and causes vertical lines to appear in this area. Fine lines gradually turn into deeper creases and furrows, when the skin in the bottom of the facial line becomes thinner and the connective collagen and elastin network of the skin deteriorates.

Massage and manual stretching

Skeletal muscles are simple to stretch just by positioning the joints in such way that the distance between the origin and insertion points of muscles running over the joints becomes greater. In the face, however, the mimic muscles covering the space between the eyebrows and in the forehead, for example, do not cross over a joint. Therefore, for anatomical reasons they, as well as many other stiffened mimic muscles of the face, need to be streched and relaxed differently. Composed of varied and safe manual stretching amd massage techniques, MimiLift Facial MuscleCare offers a comfortable solution to this as the techniques are easy to learn and can be performed independently.

MimiLift relaxing procedures apply force through longitudinal, cross-wise or twisting actions and pressure that penetrates the surface of the skin, thus remoulding the underlying mimic muscles. The multidirectional stretching relieves stiffness in the whole facial myofascial system, improves muscle elasticity and smooths out lines and creases. MimiLift relaxing techniques also make us more aware of any tensions we hold in our facial muscles, thus enabling us to avoid unnecessarily straining our face.

PRACTICAL APPLICATIONS
OF MIMILIFT FACIAL REJUVENATION

MimiLift facial rejuvenation is a combination of procedures. These are strengthening of the lax structures to lift the features and prevent facial sagging, building of the muscle tissues to provide fullness to the face and releasing and relaxing layers of facial muscles and connective tissue to diminish facial lines and creases.

Lift your face and smooth facial lines

Facial ageing is not just about skin wrinkling. Wrinkles can be seen in even relatively young people who have spent too much time in the sun without proper UV protection. Yet there are other factors that contribute to the aged look at least as much as wrinkles, and these are changes in the shape of face and deep facial lines and furrows.

As we age, the natural tendency of muscles is to atrophy and become lax, and this includes the facial area. This contributes to facial sag, droopiness and an aged look.

When the mimic muscles tighten, the taut mimic muscles will pull the overlying skin into pleats, resulting gradually in permanent facial lines and creases.

MimiLift facial rejuvenation procedures focus on prevention and reduction of facial sagging and facial lines and creases. Here are examples of how to treat to most common muscle-based ageing changes in the face. The detailed instructions are found in Chapter 5. Enjoy your natural facial rejuvenation with MimiLift!

1 Smoothing horizontal lines on the forehead
Procedure: Relaxing the frontalis muscles.

2 Smoothing horizontal and vertical creases between the eyebrows
Procedure: Relaxing the corrugator supercilii, depressor supercilii and procerus muscles.

3 Smoothing radial lines around the eyes
Procedure: Relaxing the orbicularis oculi muscle.

4 Smoothing radial lines around the lips
Procedure: Relaxing the orbicularis oris muscle.

5 Smoothing nose to mouth creases
Procedure: Relaxing all the muscles that raise the corner of the mouth and the upper lip.

6 Smoothing lines going down from the corners of the mouth, chin crease and raising the corners of mouth that tighten downwards
Procedure: Relaxing the depressor anguli oris, depressor labii inferioris, platysma and mentalis muscles. Strengthening the muscles that raise the corner of the mouth.

7 Plumping both lips
Procedure: Remoulding the orbicularis oris muscle with relaxing and strengthening exercises.

8 Lifting the eyebrows and upper eyelids
Procedure: Strengthening the frontalis muscle and the upper part of orbicularis oculi muscle. Relaxing the lateral part of the orbicularis oris muscle and the muscles between the eyebrows.

9 Lifting and adding fullness to the upper cheeks and midface
Procedure: Strengthening all the muscles that lift the corner of the mouth and the upper lip. Relaxing the chewing muscles in the cheek area.

10 Toning the lower cheek
Procedure: Strengthening the buccinator and risorius muscles. Relaxing the platysma muscle.

INSTRUCTIONS

- The combination of MimiLift voluntary strengthening exercises and functional electrical facial muscle stimulation offers an extremely effective natural facelift, making the face look firmer, filled, lifted and more toned.

- Both voluntary and electrostimulated strengthening facial exercises must be balanced with relaxing MimiLift massage and stretching procedures in order to avoid excessive tightening of the facial musculature. For example, if you strengthen your forehead's muscle for a brow lift, you also need to remould it with massage in order to prevent and reduce horizontal forehead creases.

- The precise upward and outward motions of the MimiLift manual stretching and massage techniques boost the skin's collagen and elastin production and improve facial blood and lymphatic circulation for a firm, glowing skin and reduction of wrinkles. High-quality skin creams such as products containing vitamin C and different forms of retinol work well with MimiLift. Anti-ageing creams can make the skin look better, but no cream can strengthen or stretch the muscles, because it is physiologically impossible.

- After relaxing a whole mimic muscle, you can concentrate on plumping out single creases and furrows by massaging and spreading them out with your fingers. Do not manipulate the same facial area too long in one session. Watch the reaction of your skin. The skin will redden a little with massage. This is a healthy, normal, temporary reaction, an obvious testament to improved blood flow, but overtreating the same spot may irritate the skin.

Extra: Removing pillow creases on your face

When you sleep on your stomach or on your side with your face pressed against a pillow for a number of hours, you may wake up with pillow creases running all over your cheeks and forehead. In older age these early morning lines in your face will take longer and longer to disappear, and they may even become permanent.

Add MimiLift procedures to your morning grooming regimen to straighten out pillow creases quickly. At first drink water in the morning just after waking up to hydrate your body. Then improve your facial blood flow by taking a short facial steam bath or by putting your face in the path of warm shower water. Finally straighten out the pillow creases by remoulding them with the help of MimiLift massage and stretching techniques. You are able to do this in less than 10 minutes and you will be ready to leave the house with a refreshed face without pillow lines imprinted on it.

MIMILIFT FACIAL REJUVENATION

All the MimiLift aesthetic procedures improve not only facial appearance, but also the health, expressiveness and vitality of your face. MimiLift Facial MuscleCare is a totally safe, reliable, completely natural, easy-to-use and inexpensive way to take care of your face. MimiLift gives you the opportunity to be a master of your own unique face.

Undertaken in one's early thirties, MimiLift Facial MuscleCare prevents the signs of premature ageing on the face. If embarked upon at a more mature age, MimiLift procedures gradually produce a more fresh and youthful appearance of the face.

MIMILIFT **NECK REJUVENATION**

Correct posture and good condition of the muscles in the neck-shoulder region greatly affect a person's appearance. MimiLift Facial MuscleCare gives you easy solutions to improve the look of your neck.

Double chin and neck creases

Fat tissue distributes unevenly in the body. The area just below the chin is a typical spot where fat cells create a local fat deposit. When the double chin is a local fat accumulation under the chin, even a young person may have it. Some people have loose, hanging skin under their chin. Major weight loss can leave excessive, sagging skin.

Poor posture with a collapsed upper body, head-forward position and raised shoulders makes the neck look shorter and the double chin more ap-

parent. The slumped upper body posture also contributes to the creation of a neck hump. Horizontal creases, bands and folds on the front of the neck are caused by the tightening of the platysma muscle.

Tapping the area under the chin with fingers does not remove or prevent double chin. The muscles moving the tongue are right under the chin, but training these muscles will not eliminate double chin, either. No self-treatment can tighten a significantly large amount of excess saggy skin hanging under the chin.

Front neck stretch

Relaxing the platysma muscle in the front of the neck diminishes neck creases and bands. The platysma muscle stretches and relaxes in neck rotations and backward bending. This is an effective platysma stretch.

a) Move your lower jaw forwards and then upwards so that you can extend your lower lip widely over your upper lip. Keep your jaw and lips like this and tilt your head slightly back. Pull the corners of your mouth towards your ears.

Hold this position for 3–5 seconds. You will feel a stretch around the jawline and in the front of your neck. You will feel more stretch in the front of your neck if you place your hands firmly right below your collarbones and press downward during the stretch.

Return your head and jaw slowly to the neutral position. Repeat 5 times.

b) You can intensify the stretch also by gently pushing the soft tissues around the jaw angle upwards with your fingers.

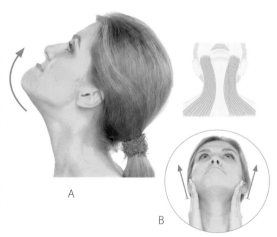

A

B

PROCEDURE: Relaxing the platysma muscle.
IMPACT ON APPEARANCE: Prevents and softens neck creases. Tones the jawline.

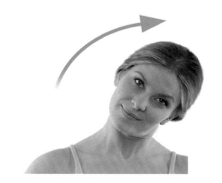

Move your neck

Good upper body posture and good condition of the muscles in the front, side and back of the neck and shoulders are the best ways to improve the appearance of your neck. Look at dancers. They generally have a great-looking and elegant neck-shoulder region. Because of their work, dancers need to keep their posture elegant and maintain wide movement in the neck, whole spine, shoulders and upper limbs.

Stretching and massage of the neck muscles and exercises that include physiologically correct neck movements will keep your neck area in shape. Detailed instructions are found in Chapter 7.

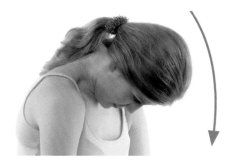

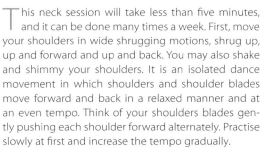

This neck session will take less than five minutes, and it can be done many times a week. First, move your shoulders in wide shrugging motions, shrug up, up and forward and up and back. You may also shake and shimmy your shoulders. It is an isolated dance movement in which shoulders and shoulder blades move forward and back in a relaxed manner and at an even tempo. Think of your shoulders blades gently pushing each shoulder forward alternately. Practise slowly at first and increase the tempo gradually.

Then bend your neck from side to side, back and forth, and rotate it by turning your head to the right and to the left. Repeat movements in each direction at least 10 times. Move your neck in a controlled way. Keep your upper posture correct, chest gently lifted, shoulders down and allow your neck to be free.

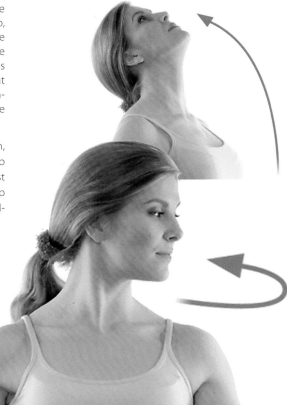

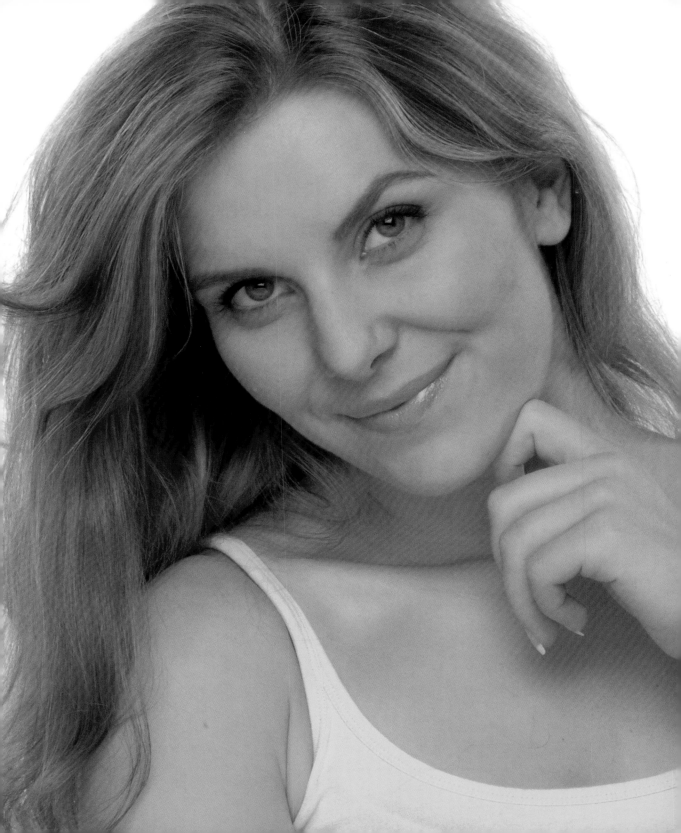

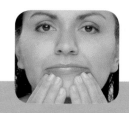

HEALTH PROBLEMS AND TREATMENTS

10

TREATMENTS FOR **TEETH CLENCHING** AND **GRINDING**

Temporomandibular disorders (TMD for short) is a medical term used to describe all functional disturbances of the chewing muscles and jaw joints. Even though the help of medical professionals is needed in most cases, good self-care plays a big role in treating TMD.

Symptoms and signs of TMD

The term temporimandibular refers to the joint, muscle and ligament connections between the temporal and mandibular bones. Temporomandibular disorders are a group of conditions that affect the chewing muscles and the jaw joints.

Myofascial pain is the most common form of TMD, meaning discomfort or pain in the muscles that control jaw functions. Because the body consists of a series of structural and neurological connections, a problem

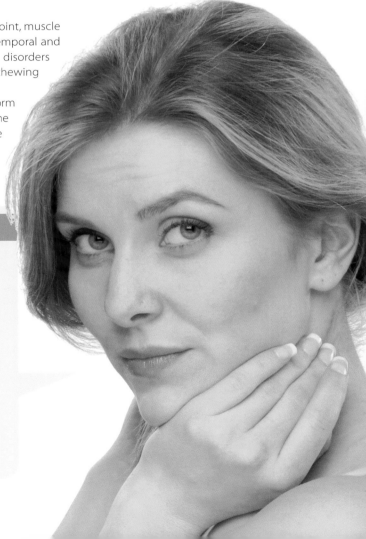

COMMON SYMPTOMS OF TEMPOROMANDIBULAR DISORDERS

- sore chewing muscles
- headaches
- stiff jaw
- jaw becomes easily fatigued when speaking or eating
- difficulties in opening the mouth wide
- pain in the jaw joint
- sensitive teeth
- unexplained pain in the face
- neck pains
- ringing and stuffiness of the ears
- earaches without infection
- a common clinical finding of the TMD is a premature wear of teeth

in the chewing muscles or in the jaw joints can cause problems in other areas of the head, spreading to the neck and even further down the shoulders and arms.

The structures of the ear are located just above the jaw joint. This close proximity explains why problems with jaw joints and chewing muscles can affect the ear.

Bruxism

Although no single cause accounts for all the symptoms and signs of TMD, bruxism plays a significant role in TMD. Bruxism is the medical term for the unconscious, nonfunctional, nonpurposeful grinding or clenching the teeth. Clenching is an intensive closing of the lower jaw and grinding is moving the jaw from side to side with the teeth in contact.

Bruxism commonly occurs during sleep. Symptoms of night-time bruxism are often a headache and stiff and sore jaw just after waking up in the morning. Most people are totally unaware of their bruxism and thus cannot link the symptoms to it.

Along with causing headaches, jaw, face and neck pains, bruxism can also damage the teeth. Because most people do not realize they have the habit, they are usually not diagnosed with bruxism until their teeth are permanently damaged.

Bruxism destroys the teeth by chipping them and wearing them down over time. Sometimes the teeth are worn down so much that the enamel is rubbed off, exposing the softer, sensitive inside of the tooth called dentin. However, the presence of tooth wear does not mean that the person is currently clenching or grinding his or her teeth. The tooth wear may have occurred many years ago.

Professional medical care for TMD

An effective dental treatment for TMD caused by bruxism is a custom-made, hard acrylic occlusal appliance, often called a bite splint, bite plate or a nightguard. An occlusal appliance will not cure the bruxism, but it can relieve the symptoms and prevent further damage to the teeth.

An occlusal splint is typically worn at night while asleep. It is designed to cover the biting surfaces of the teeth in one of the jaws, usually the upper jaw. An occlusal appliance prevents the back teeth from coming into contact and the teeth from grinding, thus providing muscle relaxation and support for the jaw joints. Permanent use of the occlusal spints may not be recommended.

TMD should always be treated extremely conservatively, using non-invasive, reversible treatments such as occlusal splints. Conservative treatments do not invade the tissues, and reversible treatments do not cause permanent, irreversible changes in the structures of the teeth or jaw joints. One form of irreversible dental treatment that is of little value, and can even worsen the problem, is grinding down the healthy teeth in an effort to try to balance the bite.

Temporomandibular disorders are typically complex. For example, there is a link between the malfunctioning of the upper neck, rigid upper thoracic spine and problems in the chewing muscles and jaw joints, for which reason a dentist alone may not be able to manage all the disorders. Treatments from other licensed health care professionals, such as physiotherapists, osteopaths and naprapaths, who are specially trained in treating temporomandibular disorders, are often needed to provide the best success for the patient suffering from TMD.

Treating TMD should be teamwork with the patient, a dentist and other treating therapists all communicating and working in the patient's best interest. The most successful recovery will be achieved when the patient actively takes part in the treatment.

Massage techniques

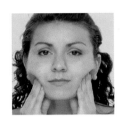

Sustained contraction of the chewing muscles initiates local muscular tenderness and even referred pain. When muscle pain is the main problem, pain relief can be achieved by manual massage. Massage mobilizes the stiff muscles, increases blood flow to the area, eliminates local soreness of the muscles and stimulates the nervous system to suppress the pain. Application of moist heat is sometimes a helpful relaxing procedure before the massage.

Once the pain is reduced, it is easier to gently and gradually stretch the chewing muscles to their normal, full length.

Stretching techniques

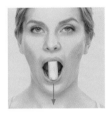
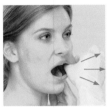

Stretching is aimed at regaining and maintaining the optimal length of the chewing muscles. Stretching restores, improves and maintains the healthy function of the chewing muscles and jaw joints in a physiologically ideal range of motion. Stretching also relieves pain and tension caused by tightened chewing muscles.

Tight, shortened chewing muscles change the rest position of the lower jaw, changing the bite. When the change of the bite is a result of a muscular disorder, the first thing to do is treat the muscles involved. Appropriate stretching lenghtens the shortened chewing muscles to allow the lower jaw to find its best resting position and to correct the bite (occlusion).

Tight chewing muscles overload and pressure the jaw joints and cause faulty movements as well as limited mouth opening. Stretching relieves the pressure and restores the normal function of the jaw joints.

Sometimes a local trauma is a side effect of a local anaesthetic injection given for dental procedures. It manifests in muscle spasms in the chewing muscles that can last several days after the treatment. Begin to relieve the muscle tension by stretching the chewing muscles very gently and carefully, not immediately but about two days after the traumatic event.

Jaw exercises

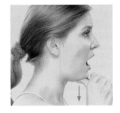

Rhythmical, delibrate use of the chewing muscles reduces muscle pain, encourages optimal healthy muscle function and condition and improves the coordinated function of the jaw joints.

Gentle, controlled jaw movements produce a growth stimulus in the cartilage of the jaw joints, reduce jaw joint pain and maintain the normal function and range of motion of the jaw joints.

Resisted jaw exercises strengthen the chewing muscles that support the jaw joints. These exercises also create a reflex muscle reaction, which relaxes the chewing muscles.

Top 10 good habits

1 Become aware and avoid bad oral habits: teeth clenching and grinding, unnecessary teeth touching or resting together, pushing tongue against teeth and tensing the jaw. Do not bite your fingernails, pens or pencils.

2 Try to find the most relaxed position of your lower jaw. The best position feels comfortable and provokes as little tension of the chewing muscles as possible.

3 Learn the proper resting position of your lower jaw: the teeth slightly apart, the lips very lightly closed and your tongue near the front teeth. The open space between the upper and lower back teeth is about 3 mm. When there is no teeth contact, the tension of the chewing muscles decreases.

4 Remember a good upper body posture with a good aligned position of the head.

5 Avoid sleeping on your stomach since it strains your jaw and neck muscles. Use a good pillow which supports the curves created by your head, neck and shoulders.

6 Breathe through your nose rather than mouth. Breathe naturally. Relax your chest and abdomen and allow them to expand.

7 Avoid excessive gum chewing.

8 Chew your food on both sides of your back teeth.

9 Do not rest your jaw on your hand.

10 Avoid exposing your head, especially the temporalis muscle, and your upper body to cold draughts.

Avoid tooth erosion

Bruxers destroy and wear their teeth by rubbing them together. Tooth erosion is another major cause of premature tooth wear, which is seen even in teenagers. Regular and prolonged exposure to acidic drinks and food is corrosive to dental enamel. Stomach acids also can cause erosion if they come up into the mouth. Both bruxism or aggressive tooth brushing will worsen the effects of erosion.

If you are sipping acidic drinks such as soft drinks, sodas, sport drinks, fruit juices or wine the whole day long, you are bathing your teeth in acid. Citric acid and phosphoric acid are the most common erosive acids found in soft drinks. The combination of hard foods and acids, such as salads with vinegar or lemon juice dressings, can be devastating to the teeth. However, there is no single food or drink that is solely responsible for dental erosion. Enjoy everything in moderation; just be aware of the effects of your diet to your dental health.

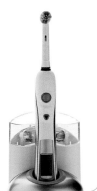

Tips to slow down dental erosion

• Rinse your mouth with water after drinking or eating something acidic.

• Avoid brushing your teeth for one hour after consuming acidic food or drink.

• Use a soft electrical tooth brush.

• Avoid excessive bleaching of your teeth.

Treatment for premature tooth wear

The best treatment is prevention. Try to protect your teeth from all forms of excessive wear. Ask your dentist to check for any signs of abnormal tooth wear and do not skip regular dental visits.

Tooth wear is often a combination of different factors – the cumulative effects of an otherwise healthy diet with a lot of nuts and hard vegetables and fruits; the present or past habit of bruxism. Whatever the reasons for tooth wear, the result is flattened, shortened teeth. Also old, worn-out fillings in the back teeth will flatten them.

Shortened teeth change the way the upper and lower teeth meet (the bite), tighten the chewing muscles and can be one of the causes behind the temboromandibular disorders. Worn-down, flattened teeth also affect the appearance. Premature flattened teeth look old and result in creasing at the corners of the mouth, thinning of the lips and premature lines around the mouth.

The teeth might be so worn down that they need to be restored. With the help of skilled restoration the teeth will regain their normal size and the jaw will regain its normal resting position. Dental restorations will improve both health of the chewing muscles and jaw joints and the appearance of the teeth, lip area and the whole lower face.

In the dentist's chair

When visiting the dentist, the more relaxed you are able to remain, the less you will tense your chewing and neck muscles during the procedures.

It is quite normal to be afraid of the dental treatments. Tell the dentist about your dental fears. A lot can be done to make the dental visits as stress-free and painless as possible. Local anaesthesia will take away feelings of pain. If you are afraid of the injection, the dentist can numb the area with a gel before inserting the needle.

Lying in a dental chair with your mouth wide open for an extensive dental procedure can overload your chewing and neck muscles. Trauma can arise from unaccustomed use, such as suddenly opening the mouth extremely wide or keeping the mouth wide open for a very long time.

So keep your mouth open in a relaxed manner and open it only as much as needed. Close your mouth and let your jaw rest for a moment whenever it is possible during the dental treatment. Try to find a comfortable position in the dental chair. Prolonged extension of the neck increases tension in the chewing muscles. If you can't find a relaxed position for your neck, do not hesitate to ask the dental staff to help you.

DENTAL FILLINGS

When the dentist has put a filling in your tooth, he always checks the ideal height of the filling. You also need to give your opinion regarding how well the filling feels to fit with your bite. It might be difficult to give a certain answer, if the local anaesthesia has numbed your mouth and your jaw area. See your dentist again if you feel any discomfort with the new filling. The filling may need to be reshaped to fit better.

To prevent any improperly occluding dental filling or crown from changing the bite and overloading the chewing muscles and jaw joints, make an appointment with your dentist as soon as possible. A missing back tooth will overload and change the bite, too. A dental implant can be used to replace the lost tooth. Before any dental procedures talk to your dentist about the treatment and possible alternatives to treat the condition.

JAW JOINT PROBLEMS AND TREATMENTS

Jaw joint problems are a part of the collection of symptoms and diseases called temporomandibular disorders. Faulty function of the chewing muscles may lead to jaw joint disturbances. Jaw exercises are essential to achieve and maintain the healthy function and mobility of the jaw joints.

Mechanical jaw joint disorders

The jaw joints are flexible and allow the lower jaw to move freely in many directions. When the lower jaw moves, the rounded ends of the lower jawbone (condyles) glide along the sockets of the temporal bones. The condyles slide back to their original position when the jaw is closed. This movement occurs inside the jaw joints. To separate the condyles from the temporal bones and to keep the movements smooth, a fibrous articular disc lies between the bones. It is attached to the head of the lower jawbone and moves with it.

If this system does not function correctly, sounds and noises may be heard from the jaw joints and the movement of the lower jawbone may be impaired. Any jaw joint symptoms and signs should be resolved as soon as they first appear.

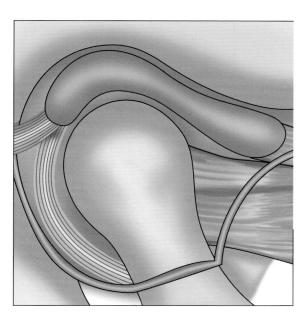

PROBLEM: Clicking jaw joints

Sometimes a clicking sound occurs upon jaw opening, closing or both. Clicking sounds from the jaw joints without painful or limited jaw opening are quite common. In a large study that followed patients over a 20-year period, joint sounds rarely progressed into a significiantly bothersome problems (Magnusson, Eagermark, Carlsson 2000).

TREATMENT: It is important that the clicking sound does not occur or occurs minimally when performing the jaw exercises. A mirror helps in learning a controlled straight downwards direction of the lower jaw without clicking sounds during the movement. The click is usually eliminated by bringing the lower jaw slightly forward and then open.

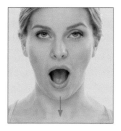

PROBLEM: ## Incorrect movements of the lower jaw

A noticeable deviation in the jaw-opening midline pathway is a typical incorrect jaw movement. Other movement problems are a catching sensation of the lower jaw and the sensation of the jaw 'going out' whenever opening it wide.

When the jaw catches and gets stuck, a person having this disorder can get the jaw back to functioning normally by moving the jaw around a little.

TREATMENT: Coordinated jaw opening exercises with the help of a hand mirror will train the straight downward direction of the lower jaw without any deviations during the movement. Moving the lower jaw in a slightly protruded position during the jaw opening will eliminate the catching sensations. Keeping the tip of the tongue against the roof of the mouth behind the front teeth while opening the jaw slowly will assist in straight and smooth jaw movement.

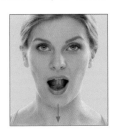

PROBLEM: ## Wide-open locked jaw

This quite rare problem is easy to diagnose – a person's jaw is locked in the wide-open position. Because a person with an open locked jaw can't tell about the problem and the pain and distress, he or she often becomes panicked. The reaction is an attempt to close the mouth, which will worsen the cramp in the chewing muscles and increase the pain.

Open locked jaw (spontaneous dislocation) is typically produced by a very wide jaw opening, such as an extended yawn or a long dental procedure. Even though open lock can occur in any jaw joints that are suddenly forced beyond their normal opening limit, some joints have an anatomical structure making them more susceptible than others to this condition.

TREATMENT: A self-help procedure is to try to open the jaw a bit more as though yawning and at the same time apply a slight backward pressure to the chin with fingers.

If this attempt does not reduce the dislocation, a visit to a hospital's emergency department is needed. The patient will be premedicated with a muscle relaxant or sedative. The physician will place his or her thumbs on the patient's back lower teeth, apply downward force on the back teeth while upward force is applied in the chin. The patient is able to close the jaw again immediately after this manipulation.

Degenerative jaw joint changes

PROBLEM: ## Osteoarthritis

Cartilage tissues of the jaw joints need a certain amount of loading to remain healthy. Movements of the jaw joints function like a pump bringing nutrients to the articular surfaces and removing waste products. Misuse of the jaw disturbs this joint homeostasis leading to thinning of the articular cartilage. Misuse, such as overloading the jaw joint due to bruxism, causes cumulative microtraumas which eventually exceed the joint's repair capacity. The articular cartilage will destruct and wear away.

In radiography, advanced osteoarthritis appears as the degeneration of the jaw joint structures and a reduced joint space. Noise of coarse crepitation may occur during the jaw movements of an osteoarthritic joint. Osteoarthritis may be associated with joint pain in rest as well as during jaw movements. However, there are people with x-rays showing the signs of osteoarthritis who have minimal if any symptoms.

TREATMENT: Overloading must be reduced by proper treatments of bruxism. Gentle, controlled jaw movements produce a growth stimulus in the cartilage of the jaw joints, reduce pain and maintain the normal functions and the range of motion of the jaw joints.

Inflammatory disorders of the jaw joint

PROBLEM: Jaw joint infections
and inflammations

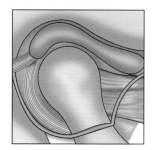

Inflammatory disorders of the jaw joints are gener- ally associated with constant, dull, aching pain in the jaw joint with possible sensations of swelling and warmth over the affected jaw joint.

Infection is caused by an invasion of infectious agents such as bacteria. Infection can spread to the jaw joints from an adjacent structure. Inflammation is not synonymous with infection. Inflammation is the body's response to tissue damage, in which the body produces chemical agents that lead to pain and swelling.

Common reasons for the inflammatory condi- tions of the jaw joints are micro- and macrotraumas. Macrotrauma is any sudden force to the jaw joint that can result in structural alterations such as blow to the chin during an accident or a fall. Cumulative microtraumas can result from jaw joint overloading associated with chronic muscle hyperactivity such as bruxism.

In systematic inflammatory arthritis such as rheu- matoid or psoriatic arthritis the jaw joints may also become involved.

TREATMENT: An infection is treated with proper medical support including antibiotic medication if bacteria is the cause. Depending on diagnosis, a short-term non-steroi- dal anti-inflammatory medication may be used in treat- ment of the inflammation.

In the acute state of inflammatory disorders the move- ments of the jaw should be temporarily restricted within as painless limits as possible.

After the acute stage gentle jaw-opening and jaw-clos- ing exercises create rhythmical movements that may reduce swelling. Short-term, 10–20 minute cold pack applications reduce the pain, swelling and reduce in- flammation.

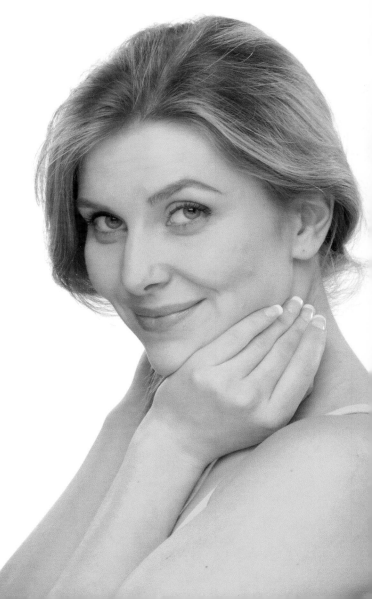

FACIAL **PALSY**

Damage to the facial nerve itself or to the brain area controlling the nerve's function can result in weakness or total loss of movement of the mimic muscles. Generally, facial palsy affects only one of the paired facial nerves, in which case only one side of the face becomes paralyzed.

Bell's palsy

Disorders of the functioning of the facial nerve can manifest themselves as facial palsy. When mimic muscles become paralyzed, they can't move and the affected half of the face becomes motionless and expressionless. A person suffering from facial palsy may not be able to lift the eyebrow on the affected side, has difficulty closing the eye and may experience drooping of the corner of the mouth.

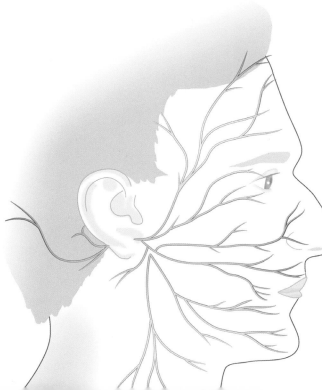

Facial functions such as eating, drinking and speaking become difficult. People with facial disfigurement as a result of facial palsy also suffer a great deal of psychological distress.

Bell's palsy is the most common form of acute facial palsy. It is named after Charles Bell, a surgeon who studied the facial paralysis 200 years ago. The term Bell's palsy is given to the conditions where the exact cause of the facial palsy is not known. Though a clear-cut reason for Bell's palsy has not yet been established, some theories suggest that reactivation of herpes viruses in the facial nerve might be responsible for the condition.

For example, it is thought that an inflammation will cause swelling in the facial nerve. When the facial nerve swells, it gets jammed in its tiny bony canal inside the skull, suffers from ischemia and becomes unable to send signals to the mimic muscles to contract. As a result, mimic muscles become paralyzed on the side of the face where the facial nerve has been affected.

Symptoms of facial palsy can range from mild to severe, from facial weakness with partial loss of voluntary facial movements (paresis) to complete loss of facial movements (paralysis) on the affected side. In complete facial paralysis strong facial asymmetry can make the face look significantly distorted.

Prognosis of Bell's palsy

Bell's palsy typically develops within a few hours or overnight. Anyone who becomes afflicted should seek medical care without delay. Bell's palsy is usually temporary and has a good recovery rate: approximately 70% of patients will have recoveries within a few weeks to a few months after onset. Even though most patients recover, recovery is sometimes incomplete and some weakness may continue or abnormal facial movement patterns may develop.

It is difficult to predict the future recovery during the first days of Bell's palsy. That is why it is important to do everything possible immediately after onset to ensure each patient reaches as complete a recovery as possible. Immediate medication and appropriately designed long-term rehabilitation carried out with dedication are notable treatments for Bell's palsy.

Medical treatment of Bell's palsy

It is necessary that a person with Bell's palsy is examined and medicated at first by a physician familiar with the disease. Treatment of acute Bell's palsy is initially medical, and medication must be undertaken without delay within two days of the emergence of symptoms.

Doctors typically prescribe oral anti-inflammatory and antiviral medication. Corticosteroids have been shown in many studies to reduce inflammation and swelling of the facial nerve, which should minimize nerve compression and damage. According to the herpes virus theory, antiviral drugs are often added to the medication to tame the herpes virus. The treatment may be enhanced by taking vitamins B, especially B 12, omega-3 fish oils and other possible dietary supplementation under the supervision of a physician.

Eye care is a very important part of treatment when a patient with Bell's palsy cannot close the eye properly. Both eye-drops which work as artificial tears and lubricant ointments keep the eye moist, thus preventing the surface of the eye from drying out. Sometimes it is necessary to wear an eye patch and tape the eye shut while asleep.

Facial palsy due to a stroke

Bell's palsy is caused by a problem in the facial nerve itself. Symptoms of facial palsy may be caused by conditions other than Bell's palsy. A serious cause is stroke. If a blood vessel in the brain gets clogged or bursts, the brain becomes damaged, and if the part of the brain that controls the function of the facial nerve is damaged, it leads to the paralysis of the muscles on one side of the face.

LEARN TO RECOGNIZE STROKE SYMPTOMS

- Sudden numbness or weakness of face, arm or leg on one side of the body. It can be a sign of a stroke if one side of the mouth suddenly droops when the person tries to smile, or if suddenly one arm begins to fall when a person tries to raise both arms over the head at the same time.
- Sudden trouble speaking and understanding simple statements, slurred speech or inability to find the words. If a person is suddenly unable to repeat a simple sentence, he or she might have had a stroke.
- Sudden trouble seeing with one or both eyes, blurred, double or blackened vision.
- Sudden trouble with walking. A person may suddenly begin to stumble or experience sudden dizziness and loss of balance or loss of coordination.
- Symptoms of a stroke are often painless, but sometimes a sudden severe headache with no apparent cause and different from previous headaches is a sign of a stroke. The headache may be accompanied by vomiting, dizziness or altered consciousness.

When a stroke is the cause of facial paralysis, the person may still be able to raise both eyebrows and close both eyes, unlike in the case of Bell's palsy. With a stroke, other muscles on the same side of the body are also involved. Stroke often spares involuntary, emotional facial movements such as spontaneous smiling, because these functions are controlled from areas of the brain that are not affected.

A person having any stroke symptoms should be taken immediately to the hospital's emergency unit in an ambulance. Every minute matters. Never just wait and see if the symptoms go away. It is normal that the symptoms may fluctuate, and it is common that there is no sensation of pain.

The earlier the treatment begins, the greater the chances are that the person having a stroke will receive treatment that can minimize the long-term consequences of the stroke. If a clot-dissolving medication is given in the case of a blood clot within three hours of the first symptoms, it may reduce long-term disability of this most common type of strokes. Ideally, the person having signs of a stroke should be in the emergency room within 60 minutes of the first symptoms.

Rehabilition of a facial palsy due to a stroke is a part of the medical rehabilitation of all the resulting disabilities. A multiprofessional team consisting of the treating neurologist and physical, speech and occupational therapists specialized in neurological rehabilitation provide a comprehensive support for the patient suffering from stroke.

Facial palsy due to a tick bite

Lyme disease is a bacterial infection which can cause facial palsy. Lyme disease got its name from the town of Old Lyme in the United States, where the disease was first reported in 1975. Everyone can get Lyme disease if bitten by a tick carrying borrelia bacteria.

Symptoms begin days or weeks after the tick bite. They are similar to the flu and there might be a little redness around the area of the bite. If not treated in the early stage, borrelia infection may spread to the nerves and joints, causing symptoms weeks to months after the initial bite. Paralysis or weakness in the muscles of the face may be one of the symptoms.

Unlike most forms of facial palsy, facial paralysis associated with borrelia infection can be prevented by early treatment with antibiotics taken in the first stage while there are only few early symptoms revealing the existence of Lyme disease.

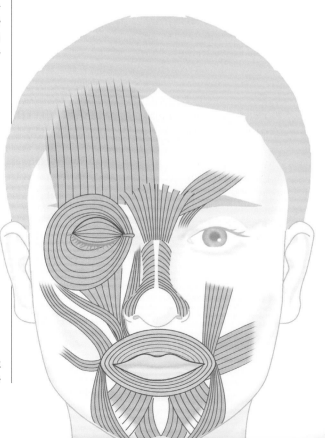

REHABILITATION OF BELL'S PALSY

Specific therapeutic facial exercises and muscle relaxation techniques support the recovery of Bell's palsy both in acute and long-term cases. Goals of rehabilition are to restore facial movements, improve facial symmetry and prevent abnormal facial mass movements.

Specialized rehabilition programme

People with Bell's palsy are typically told to do nothing and wait for the condition to get better spontaneously. Unfortunately, a complete recovery will not always occur on its own. **A specific physiotherapeutic programme consisting of isolated facial movements, facial stretching and massage techniques and relaxing exercises** has been shown to promote the recovery. Rehabilitation improves facial function even in cases of longstanding palsy.

Non-specific instructions for gross facial exercises, such as close your eyes as hard as you can, are an example of not only ineffective but even harmful methods for treating facial palsy. The wrong kind of facial exercises or wrong type of electrical stimulation to attempt to use the maximum effort to force the paralyzed muscles to move will reinforce abnormal movement patterns.

The rehabilitation of Bell's palsy is very different from common facial exercises. **It is a systematic relearning and developing process of facial movements and movement control strategies.** The objective is to learn to engage, in an appropriate manner, only the muscles required for the action and to keep other muscles relaxed.

Facial nerve-to-muscle action restores gradually. The nerve heals slowly and the regeneration can continue for many months, probably even longer. People with Bell's palsy need to give themselves time to heal and avoid hurry and any excess strain when performing the exercises.

For guidance concerning the most suitable individual rehabilitation programme it is recommended to contact a highly skilled and experienced physiotherapist specializing in facial neuromuscular rehabilitation. A professional therapist may be hard to find, because most therapists have received no specialized training in this field. Active patient participation plays the most important role in the rehabilitation process. Although each patient's programme may differ, here are general rehabilitation guidelines for Bell's palsy.

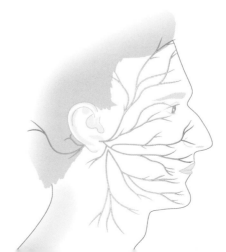

BASIC EXERCISES

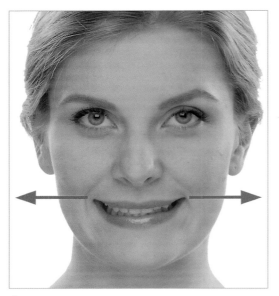

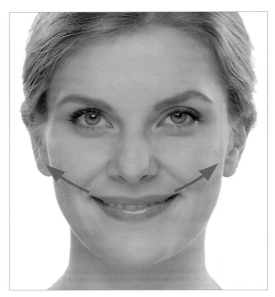

1 Pull the corners of your mouth straight to the side.

2 Pull the corners of your mouth towards your ears, as when smiling without showing teeth.

Studying and imaginary training

Bell's palsy is a trauma to the facial nerve. During the first 10 to 14 days after the onset, let the nerve start its healing and do not try to exercise the affected side. Begin the rehabilation process by studying the facial muscles, where they are located and what movements each muscle produces. Become familiar with the facial movements by watching and feeling the movements of the uninvolved side of your face.

During this period do mental facial exercises. Remember the feeling of the movements of the healthy side. Look at pictures of the basic facial movements. Imagine that you are slowly doing the same correct symmetrical facial movements. Repeat every imaginery action 10 times, in a few sessions each day.

Small active facial movements

Active facial exercises are undertaken when clear signs of restored muscle action in the face emerge. All exercises must be carried out gently, carefully and most of all slowly. At the beginning of rehabilitation do only very small facial movements.

Imagine the correct facial movements before you actively perform them. Concentrate on the movements. A certain amount of visual feedback during the performance of exercises is useful. Check occasionally that the movements are correct by using a hand-held mirror. Limit the time spent looking in the mirror, because looking at an abnormal facial appearance may only increase the psychological distress.

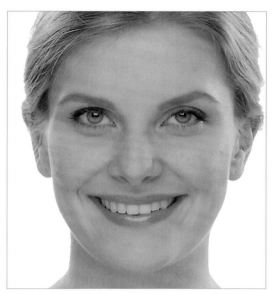

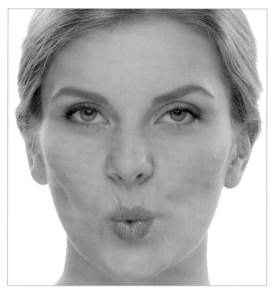

3 Pull the corners of your mouth towards your ears, as when smiling with showing teeth.

4 Pucker your lips as if whistling.

Exercise in short sessions. Do about 10 repetitions of each exercise and repeat the whole routine at least twice daily. Quality of the movements matters most. Do only as many repetitions as you can perform correctly. Avoid muscular fatigue of the involved side.

Assisted facial movements

At the beginning, the desired movement can be gently guided by the hand. For example, with the soft touch of your finger you can assist the corner of your mouth into a smiling position. Take the finger slowly off while trying to actively hold the smiling posture for a moment. Concentrate on using the appropriate muscles on the cheek area. Return the corner of the mouth slowly to the starting position.

Assist the raising of the eyebrow by gentle lifting with your finger from under the eyebrow. Take the finger off slowly while concentrating on using the forehead muscle to keep the eyebrows up for a moment. Lower the eyebrows slowly.

Full-range facial movements

Increase the range of motion and vary a little the speed of the movements only in the later stages, when the small movements can be performed without any unwanted facial movements.

Avoid unnecessary movements, such as drawing your eyebrows together or clenching your teeth.

BASIC EXERCISES

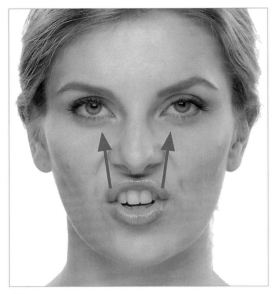

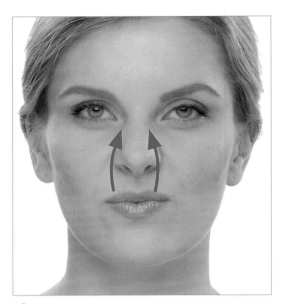

5 Raise your upper lip.

6 Raise your upper lip without showing teeth.

Resisted facial movements

In the later stages of rehabilitation, after the active range of motion is increased and no faulty facial movements exist, you can add resisted exercises to the programme. Use your fingers to carefully resist the desired facial movements. The manual resistance is applied into the opposite direction of the actual movement. The resistance subtly resists the active movement without stopping it.

Use a good range of motion. Keep the muscular movements smooth, slow and isolated. You can increase the number of repetitions to 20 and perform the session once or twice a day. Resisted exercises for mimic muscles are found in Chapter 5.

Keep facial movements symmetrical

It is important to maintain symmetry in the facial exercises. You can avoid overpowering the uninvolved facial muscles if you keep the movements small enough and concentrate on the symmetry of the movements. Diminish the movement on the affected side immediately when the muscles of the uninvolved side attempt to dominate.

Imagining the centreline of your face may help. For example, when you are pulling the corners of the mouth to the position of a smile, the lip centre is not shifted and the movement is equal in both sides of the face.

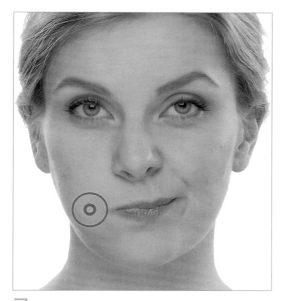

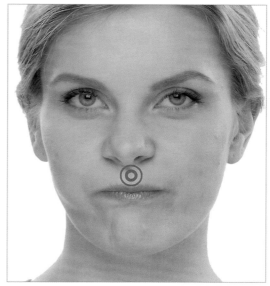

7 Puff out your cheek.

8 Puff out your upper lip.

Keep facial movements isolated

Bell's palsy changes the physiological mechanisms of the facial nerve and facial musculature in two ways. First the muscles in the affected side become weak and flaccid. In addition to paralysis of the mimic muscles, synkinesis or mass movements may develop another type of problem.

Synkinesis means simultaneous movement, an involuntary movement of muscles accompanying a voluntary movement. Synkinesis often has some predictable patterns. For example, the eye tends to close or twitch when the person with Bell's palsy tries to smile, or the corner of the mouth turns downward when trying to smile.

Focus on isolated, coordinated facial movements. Pay attention to your face as you work your mouth and eye area. For example, when you close your eyes, do not let your mouth move. Practise speaking by articulating softly and slowly all the vowels and consonants while keeping the area of the eyes relaxed.

If a synkinetic movement appears, maintain the primary movement while releasing the synkinetic muscle area. After this has been achieved, slowly return the primary movement.

BASIC EXERCISES

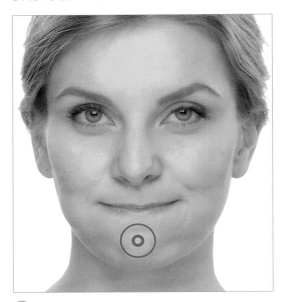

9 Puff out your lower lip.

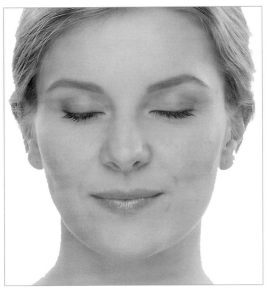

10 Gently open and close your eyes.

Stretching and massage techniques

Facial muscles of the Bell's palsy side tighten and shorten secondary to the abnormal patterns of movement called synkinesis. Tigthness and even muscle spasms may occur. The stretching techniques aim to reduce the increased muscle tonus and to relax the overactive or uncoordinated muscles in the areas of eye, cheek, mouth, chin and the front of the neck.

Massage techniques prevent stiffness, tightness and spasms of affected facial muscles and relieve the mimic muscles involved in synkinesis. Massage and stretching techniques also relax the muscles of the uninvolved side, so massage and stretch both sides of your face. Suitable relaxing procedures for mimic muscles are found in Chapter 5.

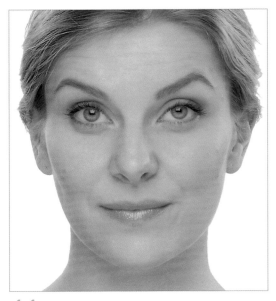

11 Lift and lower your eyebrows.

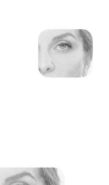

ABOUT THE AUTHOR

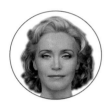

Leena Kiviluoma is a Finnish physiotherapist, engaged in teaching and expert consultation services in the fitness, beauty, health and rehabilitation industries, and editor and author of publications in the field. Her clients have included the Finnish National Opera, the Finnish National Theatre, the Parliament of Finland, Nokia and in many other companies. Numerous Finnish magazines, newspapers and TV and radio channels have published her professional advice about health and beauty.

Leena Kiviluoma began to develop MimiLift Facial MuscleCare in 1990. Her first book and video about the subject was published in Finland in 2005, and the second in 2009. Both of the products have published in other languages and have been in the 10 top-selling books of their genre.

At the request of healthcare and beauty professionals Leena Kiviluoma has started to provide courses about MimiLift Facial MuscleCare in order to give professionals new techniques to treat the facial musculature.

www.leenakiviluoma.com

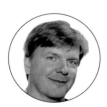

DESIGNER OF THE BOOK

Risto Kurkinen is a graphic designer with a master of arts from the University of Art and Design Helsinki. He is the illustrator, photographer and designer of the layout of all the MimiLift Facial MuscleCare products. Risto designs books and book covers for both Finnish and worldwide markets. He is a multi-skilled graphic designer, working in the varied fields of book and magazine design, as well as packaging and web design.

www.ristokurkinen.com

BIBLIOGRAPHY

A

Aalberg, Veikko, Partinen, Markku: *Päänsärky ja sen hoito.* Recallmed 1992.

Aalto, Anna-Liisa, Parviainen, Kati: *Auta ääntäsi.* Otava 1998.

Acland, Robert D: *Anatomian Videoatlas. Ihmisen anatomia. Pää ja niska, osa 1.* (Suom. Silvennoinen, Silja, Ylinen, Jari, Haarala, Risto) Medirehab kustannus 1996.

Acland, Robert D: *The Video Atlas of Human Anatomy. The Head and Neck, Part 2.* Lippincott Williams & Wilkins 1996.

Alaranta, Hannu, Pohjolainen, Timo, Rissanen, Paavo, Vanharanta, Heikki: *Fysiatria.* Duodecim 1997.

Alexeyev, Mikhail F, LeDoux, Susan P, Wilson, Glenn L: *Mitochondrial DNA and aging.* Clinical Science 2004; 107: 335–364.

Al-Majed, A A, Brushart, T M, Gordon, T: *Electrical stimulation accelerates and increases expression of BDNF and trkB in regenerating rat femoral motoneurons.* Eur J Neurosci. 2000; 12(12):4381–90.

Al-Majed, A A, Neumann, Catherine M: *Brief Electrical Stimulation Promotes the Speed and Accuracy of Motor Axonal Regeneration.* The Journal of Neuroscience 2000; 20(7):2602–2608.

Antell, D E, Taczanowski, E M: *How environment and lifestyle choices influence the aging process.* Annals of plastic surgery 1999; 43(6):585–588.

Antell, D E, Orseck, Michael J: A *Comparison of Face Lift Techniques in Eight Consecutive Sets of Identical Twins.* Plastic and Reconstructive Surgery 2007; 120(6):1667–1673.

Arponen, Ritva, Airaksinen, Olavi: *Hoitava hieronta.* WSOY 2001.

B

Barsade, Sigel G: *The Ripple Effect: Emotional Contagion and its Influence on Group Behavior.* Administrative Science Quarterly 2002; 47(4):644–675.

Beal, Flint M: *Mitochondria take center stage in aging and neurodegeneration.* Annals of Neurology 2005; 58(4):495-505.

Berk, L S, Tan, S A, Fry, W F, Napier, B J, Lee, J W, Hubbard, R W, Lewis, J E, Eby, W C: Neuroendocrine and stress hormone changes during mirtful laughter. The American Journal of the Medical Sciences 1989; 298(6):390–396.

Beurskens, Carien H G, Heymans, Peter G, Oostendorp, Rob A B: *Stability of Benefits of Mime Therapy in Sequelae of Facial Nerve Paresis During a 1-Year Period.* Otology & Neurology 2006; 27(7):1037–1042.

Beurskens, Carien H G, Heymans, Peter G: *Mime therapy improves facial symmetry in people with long-term facial nerve paresis: A randomised controlled trial.* Australian Journal of Physiotherapy 2006; 52:177–183.

Beurskens, Carien H G, Heymans, Peter G: *Positive Effects of Mime Therapy on Sequelae of Facial Paralysis: Stiffness, Lip Mobility and Social and Physical Aspects of Facial Disability.* Otology & Neurology 2003; 24(4):677–681.

Beurskens, C H, Heymans, P G: *Physiotherapy in patients with facial nerve paresis: description of outcomes.* American Journal of Otalaryngology 2004; 25(5):394–400.

Browner, Waren S, Kahn, Arnold J, Ziv, Eld, Reiner, Alexander P, Oshima, Junko, Cawthon, Richard M, Hsueh, Wen Chi, Cummings, Steven R: *The genetics of human longevity.* The American Journal of Medicine 2004; 117(11):851–860.

C

Cailliet, Rene: *Head and Face Pain Syndromes.* F.A Davis Company 1992.

Carr, Janet H., Shepherd, Roberta B: *Toispuolihalvauspotilaan liikkeiden uudelleenoppiminen.* Valtion painatuskeskus 1989.

Cederwall, E., Olsen, MF, Hanner, P, Fogdestam, I: *Evaluation of a physiotherapeutic treatment intervention in Bell's facial palsy.* Physiother Theory Pract. 2006 Jan; 22(1):43–52.

Clarkson, Hazel M: *Musculoskeletal assessment.* Lippincott Williams & Wilkins 2000.

Clay, James H, Pounds, David M: *Basic Clinical Massage Therapy.* Lippincott Williams & Wilkins 2003.

Cleland, Joshua A, Palmer, Jessica A: *Effectiveness in Manual Physical Therapy, Therapeutic Exercise, and Patient Education on Bilateral Disc Displacement without Reduction of the Temporomandibular Joint: A Single-Case Design.* Journal of Orthopedic & Sports Physical Therapy 2004; 34(9):535–548.

Cosgrove, Maeve C, Franco, Oscar H, Granger, Stewart P, Murray, Peter G, Mayes, Andrew E: *Dietary nutrient intakes and skin-aging appearance among middle-aged American women.* American Journal of Clinical Nutrition 2007; 86(4):1225–1231.

Brushart, Thomas M, Hoffman, Paul N, Royall, Richard M, Murinson, Beth B, Witzel, Christian, Gordon, Tessa: *Electrical Stimulation Promotes Motoneuron Regeneration without Increasing Its Speed or Conditioning the Neuron.* The Journal of Neuroscience 2002; 22(15):6631–6638.

Byron, Kristin, Terranova, Sophia, Nowicki, Stephen Jr: *Nonverbal Emotion Recognition and Salespersons: Linking Ability to Perceived and Actual Success.* Journal of Applied Social Psychology 2007; 37(11):2600–2619.

Cronin, Gaye, Steenerson, Ronald Leif: *The effectiveness of neuromuscular facial retraining combined with electromyography in facial paralysis rehabilitation.* Otolaryngology and Head and Neck Surgery 2003; 128:534–538.

Dimberg, Ulf: *Facial Reactions to Facial Expressions.* Psychophysiology 1982; 19(6):643–647.

D

De Laat, Antoon, Stappaerts, Karel, Papy, Sven: *Counseling and physical therapy as treatment for myofascial pain of the masticatory system.* Journal of Orofacial Pain 2003; 17(1):42–49.

E

Engström, Mats, Berg, Thomas, Stjernquist-Desatnik, Anna, Axelsson, Sara, Pitkäranta, Anne, Hultcrantz, Malou, Kanerva, Mervi, Hanner, Per, Jonsson, Lars: *Prednisolone and valaciclovir in Bell's palsy: A randomised, double-blind, placebo-controlled, multicentre trial.* Lancet Neurology 2008; 7(11):976–997.

Eriksson, Lars, Bjornland, Tore: *Akuutit leukanivelongelmat.* Suomen Hammaslääkärilehti 2005; 12(4)182–189.

F

Felber, Eric S: *Botulinum toxin in primary care medicine.* Journal of the American Osteopathic Association 2006; 106(10):609-614.

Fisher, Gary J, Datta, Subhash C, Talwar, Harvinder S, Wang, Zeng-Quan, Varani, James, Kang, Semon, Voorhees, John J: *Molecular basis of sun-induced premature skin ageing and retinoid antagonism.* Nature 1996; 379:335–339.

Forssell, Heli: *Kasvokipu – komplisoitunut ongelma.* Duodecim 2004; 120(17):2073–2078.

Freeman, M. Sean: *Transconjunctival Sub-Orbicularis Oculi Fat (SOOF) Pad Lift Blepharoplasty.* Archive of Facial Plastic Surgery 2000; 2:16–21.

Freilinger, Gerhard, Happak, Wolfgang, Burggasser, Georg, Gruber, Helmut: *Facial paralysis.* Plastic Surgery; 1:157–160. Elsevier Science Publishers 1992.

Furto, Eric S, Cleland, Joshua A, Whitman, Julie M, Olson, Kenneth A: *Manual physical therapy interventions and exercise for patients with temporomandibular disorders.* Cranio: The Journal of Craniomandibular Practice 2006; 24(4):283–291.

Färkkilä, Markus, Juntunen, Juhani, Saarinen, Päivi: *Käytännön neurologia.* Recallmed 1999.

Färkkilä, Markus, Kallela, Mikko, Harno, Hanna: *Mitä uutta migreenin tutkimuksessa ja hoidossa tapahtuu.* Kansainvälinen aivoviikko 13.–19.3.2006.

G

Garanhani, Márcia Regina, Jefferson Rosa Cardoso, de Mello, Alexandra, Capelli, Guides Ribeiro, Mara Claudia: *Exercises, bell's palsy, facial paralysis, physical therapy techniques.* Brazilian Journal of Otorhinolaryngology 2007; 73(1):112–5.

Gavish, A, Winocur, E, Astandzelov-Nachmias, T, Gazit, E: *Effect of controlled masticatory exercise on pain and muscle performance in myofascial pain students: A pilot study.* Cranio: The Journal of Craniomandibular Practice 2006; 24(3):184–90.

Ghassemi, A, Prescher, A, Riediger, D, Axer, H: *Anatomy of the SMAS revisited.* Aesthetic Plastic Surgery 2004; 28(2):123–4.

H

Haanpää, Maija, Kivipelto, Leena, Pohjola, Juha, Sintonen, Harri, Hernesniemi, Juha: *Pään alueen neuralgisten kipujen hoito.* Duodecim 2005; 121:687–695.

Halsas-Lehto, Anna-Liisa, Härkönen, Anni, Raivio, Taina: *Ihonhoito kauneudenhoitoalalle.* WSOY 2005.

Headey, B, Muffels, R, Wagner, G: *Choices which change life satisfaction: Revising SWB theory to account for change.* Discussion paper series, Forschunginstitut zur Zukunft der Arbeit, No. 4953, htpp://hdl.handle.net/10419/36874. 2010.

Helkimo, Martti: *Hammaslääkärin rooli kasvojen alueen kivun hoidossa.* Suomen Hammaslääkärilehti 2005; 12(12):715–718.

Hietanen, Jari K: *Havaintoja kasvoista.* Psykologia 2001; 4:257–268.

Holland, N J, Weiner, G M: *Recent developments in Bell's palsy.* British Medical Journal 2004; 329:553–557.

Hwang, K, Jin, S, Chung, I H: *Innervation of the procerus muscle.* Journal of Craniofacial Surgery 2006; 17(3):484–486.

Härmä, Mikko, Sallinen, Mikael: *Univaje terveysriskinä.* Duodecim 2000; 116(20):2267–2273.

I

Ito, Junji, Moriyama, Hiroshi, Shimada, Kazuyuki: *Morphological Evaluation of the Human Facial Muscles.* Okijamas Folia Anatomica Japonica 2006; 83(1):7–14.

K

Kallela, Mikko: *Mitä uutta migreenin patofysiologiasta ja genetiikasta?* Duodecim 2005; 121(6):665–674.

Kalliopuska, Mirja: *Psykologian sanat.* Psykologiatutkimus 1994.

Kanerva, Mervi, Pitkäranta, Anne: *Perifeerinen kasvohalvaus.* Duodecim 2006; 122:2267–2274.

Kanerva, Mervi: *Peripheral facial palsy: Grading, Etiology and Melkersson-Rosenthal Syndrome.* Doctoral dissertation. University of Helsinki 2008.

Kirveskari, Pentti: *Bruksismi.* Duodecim 2006; 122(6):678–683.

Korhonen, Marko: *Liikunta ja vanheneminen. Ajankohtaiset tutkimushaasteet.* Liikuntatieteiden päivät 2008.

Kovero, Outi: *The effect of violin and viola playing on bony facial structures and on frequency of temporomandibular disorders.* Doctoral dissertation. University of Helsinki 1997.

Kunnamo, Ilkka, Alenius, Heidi, Hermanson, Elina, Jousimaa, Jukkapekka, Teikari, Martti, Varonen, Helena (toim.): *Lääkärin käsikirja.* Duodecim 2006.

L

Laaksonen, Satu, Erälinna, Juha Pekka, Falck, Björn: *Vitamiinitko vaaraksi.* Duodecim 2001; 117(2):180–182.

Lagus, Heli, Vuola, Jyrki: *Keinotekoiset ihon korvikkeet.* Duodecim 2004; 120(16):1977–1985.

Laiho, Marikki, Saksela, Eero: *Perimän vauriot, vanheneminen ja syöpä, erottamaton kolmikko.* Duodecim 2007; 123:1535–1536.

Larrabee, Wayne F, Makielski, Jr, Kathleen H, Henderson, Jenifer L: *Surgical Anatomy of the Face.* Lippincott Williams & Wilkins 2004.

Lindgren, Karl-August (toim.): TULES. *Tuki- ja liikuntaelinsairaudet.* Duodecim 2005.

Lipham, William J: *Cosmetic and Clinical Applications of Botox and Dermal Fillers.* SLACK Incorporated 2008.

Lockley, John: *Päänsäryt.* WSOY 1996.

Loikkanen, Aki: *H-limit.* Pansana kustannus 2006.

Lozano, Rodríguez F J, Yuguero, Sáez M R, Fenoll, Bermejo A: *Bruxism related to violin playing.* Medical problems of Performing Artists 2008; 23(1):12.

M

MacDonald, Michael R, Spiegel, Jeffrey H, Raven, Raymond B, Kabaker, Sheldon S, Maas, Corey S: *An anatomical approach to glabellar rhytids.* Archives of Otalaryngology – Head & Neck Surgery 1998; 124:1315–1320.

MacKenzie, I C, Dabelsteen, Sally: *Suun limakalvon ja syövän kantasolut.* Suomen Hammaslääkärilehti 2006; 13(4):188–193.

Magnusson, T, Egermark, I, Carlsson, G E: *A longitudinal epidemiologic study of signs and symptoms of temporomandibular disorders from 15 to 35 years of age.* Journal of Orofacial Pain 2000; 14(4):310–319.

Mandikan, N: *Effect of facial neuromuscular re-education on facial symmetry in patients with Bell's palsy: A randomized controlled trial.* Clinical Rehabilitation 2007; 21(4):338.43.

Matsumoto, David, Willingham, Bob: *Spontaneous facial expressions of emotion of congenitally and noncongenitally blind individuals.* Journal of Personality and Social Psychology 2009; 96(1):1–10.

McCarberg, Bill, O´Connor, Annie: *A new look at heat treatment for pain disorders, Part 1.* APS Bulletin 2004; 14(6).

Michelotti, A, Steenks, M H, Farella, M, Parisini, F, Cimino, R, Martina, R: *The additional value of home physical therapy regimen versus patient education only for treatment of myofascial pain of the jaw muscles: Short-term results of a randomized clinical trial.* Journal of Orofacial Pain 2004; 18(2):114–125.

Michelotti, A, Wijer, A, Steenks, M, Farella, M: *Home-exercise regimes for the management of non-specific temporomandibular disorders.* Journal of Oral Rehabilitation 2005; 32(11):779–785.

Mir, M Afzal: *Atlas of Clinical Diagnosis.* Saunders 2003.

Molteni, Raffaella, Zheng, Jun-Qi, Ying, Zhe, Gòmez Pinilla, Fernando, Twiss, Jeffery L: *Voluntary exercise increases axonal regeneration from sensory neurons.* Experimental Neurology 2008; 211(2):489–493.

Moore, Keith L: *Clinically Oriented Anatomy.* Williams & Wilkins 1992.

Moore, Keith L: *Plastic Surgery Vol. 1 & 2.* Elsevier Science Publishers B.V 1992.

Muehlberger, T, Fischer, P, Lehnhardt, M: *The anatomy of the surgical treatment of migraine.* Zentralblatt für Chirurgie 2005; 130(4):288–292.

Mustajoki, Pertti, Saha, Heikki, Sane, Timo (toimittajat): *Potilaan tutkiminen.* Duodecim 2005.

N

Netter, Frank H: *Atlas der Anatomie des Menschen.* ICON Learning Systems 2000.

Nienstedt, Walter (päätoim.): *Lääketieteen termit.* Duodecim 2005.

Nienstedt, Walter, Hänninen, Osmo, Arstila, Antti, Björkqvist, Stig-Eyrik: *Ihmisen fysiologia ja anatomia.* WSOY 1995.

Nordström, Rolf E. A: *Esteettinen kirurgia.* Otava 2001.

Nordström, Sixten: *Kaikki musiikista.* WSOY 1997.

O

Oberdoerffer, Philipp, Michan, Shaday, McVay, Michael, Mostoslavsky, Raul, Vann, James, Park, Sang-Kyu, Hartlerode, Andrea, Loerch, Patrick, Wright, Sarah M, et al: *SIRT 1 redistribution on chromatin promotes genomic stability but alters gene expression during aging.* Cell 2008; 135(5):907–918.

Ohtake, Patricia J, Zafron, Michelle L, Poranki, Lakshmi G, Fish, Dale R: *Does electrical stimulation improve motor recovery in patients with idiopathic (Bell) palsy?* Physical Therapy 2006; 86(11):1558–1564.

Oikarinen, Aarne: *Steroidien vaikutus sidekudokseen.* Duodecim 2000; 116(22):2474–2482.

Okeson, Jeffrey P: *Management of Temporomandibular Disorders and Occlusion.* Mosby Elsevier 2008.

Ozsoy, Z, Gözu, A, Genc, B: *Two-plane injection of botulinum exotoxin A in glabellar frown lines.* Aesthetic Plastic Surgery 2004; 28(2):114–115.

P

Paakkari, Ilari: *Lääkkeiden annostelu ihon kautta – riittääkö laastareille paikkoja?* Duodecim 1993; 109(20):1867.

Pageon, H, Asselineau, D: *An in vitro approach to the chronological aging of skin by glycation of the collagen.* Annals of the New York Academy of Sciences 2005; 1043:529–32.

Pageon, H, Bakala, H, Monnier, VM, Asselineau, D: *Collagen glycation triggers the formation of aged skin in vitro.* European Journal of Dermatology 2007; 17(1):12–20.

Pageon, H, Techer, M P, Asselineau, D: *Reconstructed skin modified by glycation of the dermal equivalent as a model for skin aging and its potential use to evaluate anti-glycation molecules.* Experimental Gerontology 2008; 43(6):584–588.

Palo, Jorma, Jokelainen, Matti, Kaste, Markku, Teräväinen, Heikki, Waltimo, Olli: *Neurologia.* WSOY 1992.

Palotie, Aarno, Anttila, Verneri, Nyholt, Dale R, Kallela, Mikko, Artto, Ville, Vepsäläinen, Salli, ym: *Consistently replicating locus linked to migraine on 10q22-q23.* American Journal of Human Genetics, online 17 April, 2008.

Palva, Tauno: *Korva-, nenä-, kurkkutautioppi ja foniatrian perusteet.* Korvatieto 1991.

Park, Jung I, Hoagland, Todd M, Park, Min S: *Anatomy of the corrugator supercilii muscle.* Archives of Facial Plastic Surgery 2003; 5:412–415.

Peterson Kendall, Florence, Kendall McCreary, Elizabeth, Geise Provance, Patricia: *Muscles Testing and Function.* Williams & Wilkins 1993.

von Piekartz, Harry J M: *Craniofacial Pain.* Butterworth Heinemann Elsevier 2007.

von Piekartz, Harry, Bryden, Lynn: *Craniofacial Dysfunction & Pain.* Butterworth Heinemann 2006.

Pietilä, Maisa, Sipilä, Kirsi, Raustia, Aune: *Purentaelimen toimintahäiriön esiintyvyys ja hoidon tarve.* Suomen Hammaslääkärilehti 2005; 12(3):90–96.

Pinola, Hanna, Sipilä, Kirsi, Raustia, Anne: *Purennan osuus purentaelimen toimintahäiriössä.* Suomen Hammaslääkärilehti 2006; 13(20):1152–1156.

Platzer, Werner: *Color Atlas of Human Anatomy, Vol.1, Locomotor System.* Georg Thieme 2004.

Porter, David, Barrill, Erin, Oneacre, Kathy, May, Benjamin D: *The effects of duration and frequency of Achilles tendon stretching on dorsiflexion and outcome in painful heel syndrome: A randomized, blinded, control study.* Foot Ankle International 2002; 23(7):619–624.

R

Raitio, Anina: *Tupakoinnin vaikutus ihoon.* Väitöskirja. Oulun Yliopisto, 2005.

Reichert, Bernhard: *Käytännön anatomia 2.* VK-Kustannus 2008.

Rexbye, Helle, Petersen, Inge, Johansens, Mette, Klitkou, Louise, Jeune, Bernard, Christensen, Kaare: *Influence of environmental factors on facial aging.* Age and Ageing 2006; 35(2):110–115.

Root, A.A, Stephens, J.A: *Organization of the central control of muscles of facial expression in man.* The Journal of Physiology 2003; 549(1):289–298.

S

Saari, K M (toim.): *Silmätautioppi.* Kandidaattikustannus 1999.

Saresvaara-Virtanen, Marjut, Ojala, Birgitta: *Nivelten ja lihasten fysioterapia.* Finnpublishers 1993.

Search, N A, Chang, E L, Vyas, N, Sorensen, B N, Weiland, J D: *Electrical Stimulation of the Paralyzed Orbicularis Oculi in Rabbit.* Neural Systems and Rehabilitation Engineering 2007;15:67–75

Sharav, Yair, Benoliel, Rafael: *Orofacial Pain & Headache.* Mosby Elsevier 2008.

Sharma, D C, Parihar, P S, Kumawat, D C, Dave, R R, Bhatnagar, H N, Bhatnagar, L K: *Duane's retraction syndrome with facial hemiatrophy (a case report).* JPMG 1990; 36(1): 51–53.

Sivenius, Juhani: *AVH-potilaan kuntoutus oikeassa paikassa ja oikeaan aikaan.* Erikoislääkäri 2007; 4:161–164.

Skillgate, Eva, Vingard, Eva, Alfredsson, Lars: *Naprapathic Manual Therapy or Evidence-based Care for Back and Neck Pain: A Randomized, Controlled Trial.* Clinical Journal of Pain 2007; 23(5): 431–439.

Soinila, Seppo, Kaste, Markku, Launes, Jyrki, Sommer, Hannu: *Neurologia.* Duodecim 2001.

Steinmetz, A, Ridder, P-H, Reichelt, A: *Craniomandibular Dysfunction and Violin Playing: Prevalence and the Influence of Oral Splints on Head and Neck Muscles in Violins.* Medical Problems of Performing Artists 2006; 21(4):183.

Suhonen, Raimo: *Järkeä kortikoidivoiteiden käyttöön.* Suomen lääkärilehti 2002; 9:1016–1018.

Surakka, Veikko: *Contagion and Modulation of Human Emotions.* University of Tampere 1998.

Surakka, Veikko: *Kasvonilmeet ja emootioiden tutkimus.* Psykologia 1996; 31:412–420.

Surakka, V, Hietanen, J K: *Facial and emotional reactions to Duchenne and non-Duchenne smiles.* International Journal of Psychophysiology 1998; 29(1):23–33.

T

Tanskanen, Minna, Mustafa, Atalay, Uusitalo, Arja: *Hapetusstressi ja antioksidanttikapasiteetti ylikuormittuneilla urheilijoilla.* 14. Liikuntalääketieteen päivät 27.–28.10.2005.

Targan, Robert S, Alon, Gad, Kay, Scott L: *Effect of long-term electrical stimulation on motor recovery and improvement of clinical residuals in patients with unresolved facial nerve palsy.* Otolaryngology – Head and Neck Surgery 2000; 122(2):246–52.

Travell, Janet G, Simons, David G: *Myofascial Pain and Dysfunction. The Trigger Point Manual. Vol. 1 The Upper Extremities.* Williams & Wilkins 1983.

Trifunovic, A, Wredenberg, A, Falkenberg, M, Spelbrink, J N, Rovio, A T, Bruder, C E, Bohlooly, Y M, Gidlöf, S, Oldfors, A, *et al.*: *Premature ageing in mice expressing defective mitochondrial DNA polymerase.* Nature 2004; 429(6990):357–0.

U

Ukkola, Veijo, Ahonen, Juhani, Alanko, Arto, Lehtonen, Timo, Suominen, Sinikka: *Kirurgia.* WSOY 2001.

Upledger, John E, Vredevoogd, Jon D: *Craniosacral Therapy.* Eastland Press 1993.

Urtamo, Annele, Takala, Esa-Pekka: *Näyttöpäätetyön ergonomian ohjeet täydentävät toisiaan.* Työ ja ihminen 2002; 16(4):323–337.

V

Valtakunnalliset *Lääkäripäivät 2009. Luentolyhennelmät.* Suomen Lääkäriliitto, Suomalainen Lääkäriseura Duodecim.

Vastamäki, Martti, Pohjolainen, Timo, Juntunen, Juhani: *Soittajan tuki- ja liikuntaelinvaivat.* Duodecim 2002; 118(15):1596–1602.

Vastamäki, Martti: *Lääketiedettä muusikon hyväksi.* Muusikko 2006; 8:14–15.

Vehmanen, Raili: *Suun terveydenhuollon teknologia.* FinOHTAn raportti 6, Stakes 1997.

Vrbova, Gerta, Hudlicka, Olga, Schaefer Centofanti, Kirstin: *Application of Muscle/Nerve Stimulation in Health and Disease.* Springer 2008.

Vrbova, Gerta, Schaefer Centofanti, Kristin, Clapham, Lorraine, McQueen, K S: *Medical & Therapeutic Applications of Ultratone Biostimulation.* Ultra Scientific Instruments Ltd 2002.

Vrbova, Gerta: *Rationale for activating nerves and muscles in patients with facial palsy with appropriate patterns of activity.* Department of Anatomy and Developmental Biology, University College Hospital, London, May 2001.

Vuori, Ilkka, Taimela, Seppo (toim.): *Liikuntalääketiede.* Duodecim 1995.

W

Weinzweig, Jeffrey: *Plastic surgery secrets.* Hanley & Belfus 1999.

Wessman, Maija, Kallela, Mikko, Kaunisto, Mari, Havanka, Hannele, Ilmavirta, Matti, Kaprio, Jaakko, Peltonen, Leena, Färkkilä, Markus, Palotie, Aarno: *Suomalaisista migreeniperheistä löytyi auralliselle migreenille altistava geenilokus.* Duodecim 2002; 118:445–447.

www.kaypahoito.fi

Y

Ylinen, Jari, Cash, Mel, Hämäläinen, Heikki: *Urheiluhieronta.* Medirehabook 1995.

Ylinen, Jari: *Manuaalinen terapia. Venytystekniikat 1.* Medirehabook 2002.

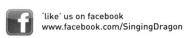
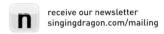
Discovering Holistic Health

Definitive guides to the key principles of a wide range of practices, these are ideal starting points for anyone wishing to explore their holistic health and wellbeing options.

Principles of Chinese Medicine

What it is, how it works, and what it can do for you
2nd Edition
Angela Hicks
Paperback: £9.99/$15.95
ISBN 978 1 84819 130 3
eIBSN 978 0 85701 113 8
224 pages

Acupuncture, Chinese herbs, qigong, tui na massage and diet therapy have been used by the Chinese for over 2000 years, and they are still the treatments of choice for millions of people throughout the East. Covering everything from the basic theory of Chinese medicine to how to find a practitioner, the book provides a definitive introductory guide to this ancient system.

Principles of Chinese Herbal Medicine

What it is, how it works, and what it can do for you
Revised Edition
John Hicks
Paperback: £9.99/$15.95
ISBN 978 1 84819 133 4
eIBSN 978 0 85701 113 8
160 pages

Covering everything from the history to the most important Chinese herbs and their properties to what to expect from a consultation, the book provides readers with all the key information about the theory and practice of this medical system.

Principles of Tibetan Medicine

What it is, how it works, and what it can do for you
Revised Edition
Dr. Tamdin Sither Bradley
Paperback: £9.99/$15.95
ISBN 978 1 84819 134 1
eIBSN 978 0 85701 114 5
224 pages

Tibetan medicine has been practised for over 2,500 years. Known as 'gSo-ba-Rig-pa', or 'the science of healing', it is based on Buddhist philosophical principles, astrology and the close relationship between body and mind. This concise introduction presents all the essential information on Tibetan medicine.

Principles of Kinesiology

What it is, how it works, and what it can do for you
Revised Edition
Maggie La Tourelle with Anthea Courtenay
Foreword by John F. Thie, D.C.
Paperback: £9.99/$15.95
ISBN 978 1 84819 149 5
eISBN 978 0 85701 119 0
200 pages

Kinesiology is a system of natural health care that combines muscle testing with the principles of Chinese medicine to assess energy and body function. This introductory guide explains how kinesiology works, how to find a practitioner and how it is usefully applied with other therapies, as well as how self-help techniques can be applied.

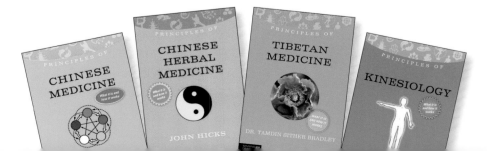

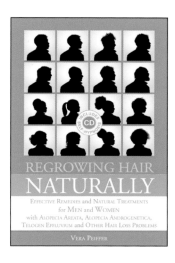

Regrowing Hair Naturally

Effective Remedies and Natural Treatments for Men and Women with Alopecia Areata,
Alopecia Androgenetica, Telogen Effluvium and Other Hair Loss Problems
Vera Peiffer

Paperback: £14.98/ $24.95
ISBN 978 1 84819 139 6
eISBN 978 0 85701 118 3
160 pages

Hair loss affects people of all ages and can be caused by a wide variety of factors. Whatever the cause of hair loss, there are natural remedies and therapies that can help the body detoxify and rebalance itself and enable healthy hair to grow again.

Containing a wealth of research and easy-to-understand tests and advice that the reader can put into practice straight away, this book covers a full range of natural approaches, from nutrition and hypnotherapy, to detoxification and bodywork exercises. There is a self-hypnosis CD included to aid stress reduction, an important factor in treating hair loss naturally.

This will be a supportive guide for anyone affected by hair loss, as well as the complementary therapists wanting to learn more about the options available for clients with hair loss problems.

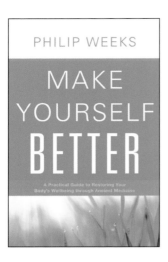

Make Yourself Better
A Practical Guide to Restoring Your Body's Wellbeing through Ancient Medicine
Philip Weeks

Paperback: £9.99/ $16.95
ISBN 978 1 84819 012 2
eISBN 978 0 85701 077 3
240 pages

Applying his deep understanding of holistic medical traditions from both East and West, Philip Weeks guides the reader through the process of restoring the body's wellbeing using a simple combination of natural techniques, diet and herbal medicines. He explores five key interconnected areas through which wellbeing can be attained – nourishment; detoxification; lifestyle; activation; and mind, emotions and spirit – based on his analogy of the wheel of health.

The author explores in depth the importance of good nutrition and detoxification, with clear explanations of specific methods and techniques and of the general principles to adhere to. He includes simple recipes and clinically tested detoxification plans. The health benefits of activity and physical exercise are explored, as are the effects of potentially harmful substances such as mercury, additives and plastics, and the simple steps that can be taken to avoid these. He also looks in a holistic way at specific emotional difficulties the reader may be faced with, such as anger, stress and grief, and at how to deal with these in order to achieve wellbeing on a mental, emotional and spiritual level.

Compassionate and realistic, *Make Yourself Better* will empower the reader to make more informed choices in their day-to-day life to achieve a greater level of health and vitality.

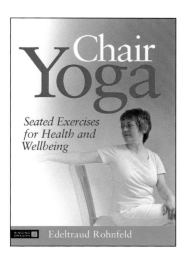

Chair Yoga
Seated Exercises for Health and Wellbeing
Edeltraud Rohnfeld
Illustrated by Edeltraud Rohnfeld

Paperback: £12.99/ $19.95
ISBN 978 1 84819 078 8
eISBN 978 0 85701 056 8
192 pages

Chair yoga is a revolutionary concept designed to make the numerous benefits of classical yoga available to a wider range of physical abilities. This step-by-step program can be practiced by virtually anyone, anywhere, in any chair, to stimulate physical and mental wellbeing.

This fully illustrated guide contains 90 easy-to-master exercises that have been specially developed for those with a limited range of movement. Clear instructions guide the reader through each routine, all of which can be carried out safely without any previous knowledge or yoga expertise. The exercises can also be adapted by yoga teachers who want to incorporate chair yoga into their classes.

This book will be popular with anyone wanting to experience the health benefits of an easy, versatile form of yoga, particularly older people, individuals rehabilitating after injury or illness and those with physical disabilities, as well as the professionals who support them.

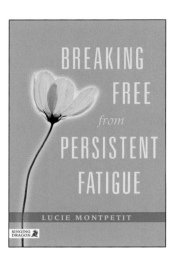

Breaking Free from Persistent Fatigue
Lucie Montpetit

Paperback: £16.99/ $24.95
ISBN 978 1 84819 101 3
eISBN 978 0 85701 081 0
288 pages

Many factors of twenty-first century life are impacting negatively on our quality of sleep and self-restorative functions. The pressure for increased productivity, less than ideal diet, constant technological changes, environmental pollution and unrealistic self-expectations mean that a growing number of people are suffering from debilitating and persistent fatigue.

This book explains the body-mind balance and how it can be destabilized resulting in fatigue. It combines practical ways to measure energy levels and identify stressors with concrete suggestions for how to modify habits, detoxify lifestyles and tackle daily challenges head on. The author employs her vast professional and personal experience of conquering myalgic encephalomyelitis (ME) to address the physiological and psychological factors affecting our energy levels, from diet and environment, to breathing and the internal workings of our bodies.

This detailed and comprehensive guide offer a fresh outlook for anyone who suffers from general fatigue, stress and conditions such as chronic fatigue syndrome, fibromyalgia, sleep disorders, adjustment disorder, depression and temporomandibular joint dysfunction as well as the professionals who work with them.

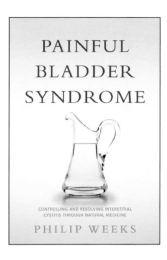

Painful Bladder Syndrome
Controlling and Resolving Interstitial Cystitis through Natural Medicine
Philip Weeks

Paperback: £13.99/ $22.95
ISBN 978 1 84819 110 5
eISBN 978 0 85701 089 6
192 pages

Painful bladder syndrome is a common and highly debilitating condition that Western medicine finds notoriously difficult to treat. Blending ancient and modern holistic medical traditions from both East and West, Philip Weeks guides the reader through the process of managing their symptoms effectively using a simple yet powerful combination of natural techniques, nutrition and herbal medicine.

Applying his deep understanding of the principles of Ayurvedic and Chinese medicine, he provides holistic medical perspectives on the causes of PBS, as well as clear explanations of specific holistic methods and techniques for bringing symptoms under control, along with step-by-step instructions for introducing them to daily life. The book also looks in a holistic way at effective natural treatments for common co-existing conditions, including allergies, fibromyalgia, irritable bowel syndrome and chronic fatigue. The book ends with an easy-to-follow seven point protocol for recovery from PBS.

This pragmatic and compassionate self-help guide will empower those with interstitial cystitis to gain control over their symptoms and achieve greater physical, emotional and spiritual wellbeing. It will also be of interest to complementary, alternative and mainstream health practitioners involved in treating or supporting those with the condition.

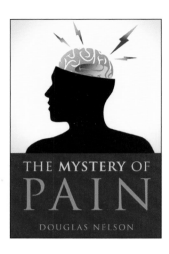

The Mystery of Pain
Douglas Nelson

Paperback: £15.99/ $25.00
ISBN 978 1 84819 152 5
eISBN 978 0 85701 116 9
224 pages

The more deeply you understand the process of pain, the more power you have to influence it. Emerging advances in the science of pain are not only fascinating; they open doors to possible avenues of treatment. This book presents a comprehensive, accessible guide to the scientific understanding of pain.

Covering the traditional scientific models of understanding as well as the current research, the book explores the different types of pain, providing clear explanations of the structures and processes involved. It examines key issues such as the placebo effect, fibromyalgia syndrome (FMS), and how social support and understanding can be powerful tools in reducing pain's devastating effects. The book also looks at diagnosis and measurement of pain, and how different models of thinking affect the relationship between patient and clinician.

Approaching pain in a practical and scientific way, the book helps readers understand the processes of pain. It will be essential reading for anyone who wants to know more about pain and pain management, alternative medicine practitioners, massage therapists and psychotherapists.